Paleo Diet
3 Books in 1 Book Set
By: Emily Simmons

Paleo Diet for Beginners

Exploring Over 20 Enticing Recipes to Energise Your Day and Excite Your Palate
By: Emily Simmons

Table of Contents

INTRODUCTION

Paleo Gluten Free Breakfast Recipes:

1. Paleo Friendly Apricot Bar for a Morning Power Boost
2. Vegetable Casserole for a Healthy Heart
3. A Quick Breakfast with a Frozen Waffle
4. Benefits of Oatmeal and Coconut in the Oatmeal
5. Stir-Fried Power Punch Bacon
6. Paleo Coconut Curry

Paleo Gluten Free Lunch Recipes:

1. The Nutrients of Cilantro Packed into Baked Lime Chicken
2. The Tangy Flavor of Spices in Tomato and Tuna Burger
3. Tasty Tostones for a Wholesome Meal
4. Joyful Jalapeno Burgers with Chicken
5. Paleo Chicken Wraps
6. Homemade Paleo Mayonnaise

Paleo Gluten Free Dinner Recipes:

1. A Great Gravy for Paleo Lovers
2. Frittata to Freshen You Up
3. Piccata with Chunky Chicken
4. Chicken with Honey Glazing
5. Zucchini Zoom Zoodles
6. Paleo Mushroom Caps

Paleo Gluten Free Desserts:

1. Paleo Vanilla Coconut Ice-Cream
2. Filled Apple Fritters
3. No-Bake Coconut Bars
4. Paleo Bites of Brownie
5. Truffles with Chocolate, Coconut and Coffee

<u>Conclusion</u>

<u>Introduction</u>

Having read the introduction, you must be wondering what is Paleo? A Paleo diet is the abbreviated form of Paleolithic diet. Yes, you got it right. It belongs to the food from the Stone Age. It is also known as the Stone Age diet or the Caveman Diet. Do you remember the Flintstones? Fred used to slog in the jungles the whole day to take care of his family. But, you do not have to ride a stone-and-wood car to fetch food from the grocery store. What do we have online shopping for? Sounds easy right? It is actually not very difficult to change your diet plan.

To explain it in the simplest of terms, the Paleo diet plan consists of only those foods which were available to our ancient ancestors such as berries, nuts and meat. It does not include foods that they were not yet familiar with, like dairy products. The period ended about 10,000 years ago with the advent of farming. But, our ancestors have given us some very valuable food lessons that we can follow for a healthy life. You do not have to go back to that age and use bone tools, stone and flint. Neither do you have to go fishing, hunting and gathering plant foods. Thank god we have supermarkets that can do this tough job for us.

Why should we follow Paleo now?

Well, the experts have the answer to this question. They say that the modern humans have maladapted themselves to eat foods like legumes, dairy and grains after the advent of agriculture. And the brownie points have been added by highly processed fast foods! The human body is not able to metabolize these foods properly, which leads to diseases such as obesity, diabetes and heart diseases. The proponents of Paleo claim that the followers of this diet may enjoy a healthier, longer and more energetic life. It is a convincing argument I guess!

What to eat in a Paleo diet?

Following a Paleo diet needs you to make a few changes in your regular diet, i.e. add a few things and remove a few things forever. Here is a list of eatables that you should welcome to your routine:

- Fish/seafood
- Grass-produced meats
- Veggies
- Fresh fruits
- Seeds and nuts
- Eggs
- Healthy oils (Walnut, Olive, Macadamia, Flaxseed, Coconut, Avocado)
- Grass-fed butter

You should exclude these things from your routine diet:

- Legumes (including peanuts)
- Cereal grains
- Refined sugar
- Dairy
- Processed foods

- Potatoes
- Refined vegetable oils
- Salt
- Fruit juices
- Processed meats
- Starchy vegetables

How can you adapt to the Paleo diet without crashing?

You must have noticed that you do not have to follow a deprived diet plan to make the transition to a Paleo diet. We will not let you crash by giving you an unrealistic diet plan. When you start shifting from a routine of processed grains to a Paleo diet, do not get intimidated. Do not deprive yourself. You will want to shift back to your normal diet if you feel hungrier. Now when you have made the good decision to shift to a Paleo diet, you should not curse yourself and instead be grateful. Follow the tips and tricks mentioned below to make your Paleo diet sustainable forever.

1. Be optimistic

You should focus on the good side of this diet. Instead of thinking that you cannot have chocolates any more, you should focus on the delicacies of the Paleo diet. There are abundant vegetables and animal proteins waiting for you.

1. Do not cheat yourself

When people start following a new diet, they generally keep a "cheat day", to cheat on the diet once a week. Don't you think that the word "cheat" itself suggests something wrong? When you keep such a day in your weekly calendar, you tend to wait for that day and that makes you feel even more deprived. The idea here is to love your Paleo food, not despise it.

1. Find out your favorite animal protein

Grass fed meat means that those animals that the meat comes from eat grass. Their meat is much healthier than carnivorous animals, i.e. which eat the flesh of other animals. Grass fed meat can get a little pricey, but still you can look for alternatives that you can afford.

1. Fat does not make people fat

It is a misconception that fat in animal meat makes you fat. Instead, an excess of sugars and carbohydrates along with fats in your diet make you fat. If you start loving fat in various forms like avocado, animal protein, nuts, seeds and coconut, you will find that you feel more energetic. Moreover, natural fat is more satiating in your meals.

1. Bring a healthy snack to the workplace

You may feel hungry after a hard day's work and thus you cannot help but stop at MacDonalds' for "just a burger". If this happens to you as well, you will end up crashing on your new diet. The healthy Paleo option is to bring a healthy snack to the workplace for evening munching so that you do not crave for "just a burger"

1. Do not include too many Paleo baked foods

Though it is fine to indulge in a few baked Paleo items once in a while, we do not recommend it that you make it a routine. Think over it logically- baking was never a principle of the Paleo diet. But since it is a need of modern-day cooking, we will teach you some baked Paleo dishes which are gluten free. If you indulge in too many Paleo muffins and ice-creams, you are missing the point. The point here is to reprogram the body to adapt to whole foods and make your body stable.

1. Do not throw away the leftovers

Our ancestors never cooked different foods for all three meals. They ate whatever they hunted and kept the leftover food for the next meal. Thus, you can eat the leftovers of morning breakfast in your lunch. And guess what! You have a refrigerator too which your Stone Age fellows never had. Wink!

1. Get support

Find some friends in your neighborhood or online who follow the Paleo diet. There are hundreds of websites, Facebook pages and blogs, where people post their experiences and Paleo diet recipes. You will enjoy having the support of some fellows who are also going through the same journey.

Paleo Gluten Free Breakfast Recipes

So now it's time to start with recipes. We will begin the healthy diet with Paleo breakfast recipes. You must have heard your mother saying that you should never skip your breakfast. And mothers are always right. Many health freaks think that skipping meals will control their weight. They jump straightaway to lunch without having any breakfast. And that's where they are wrong.

Why should you have breakfast?

Having a sumptuous breakfast is the key to good health and balanced body weight. Your efficiency at your workplace is doubled when your mind is not thinking about the lunch in your Tiffin. Leaving home without breakfast is like igniting a car without a drop of petrol. How can your body function properly after the long night hours of empty stomach?

Think of a situation when you did not have your breakfast one day and felt badly hungry till the lunch time. You must have felt like eating double your normal diet at lunch. That's the point we are making. People who skip breakfast tend to eat more at meals and throughout the day as well. Thus, they weigh more than normal.

You must have your morning meal within two hours of your waking. It will give you an edge over your friends. Here, we are talking about the Paleo breakfast. You might miss the breads and tacos you used to have. But, we will give you some amazingly delicious breakfast substitutes which will not let you miss your earlier routine.

You will be happier, healthier and more energetic than ever before once you habitually use the Paleo diet plan. This diet makes you feel lighter and more active. So let us start with the amazing delicacies of a Paleo breakfast.

Paleo Friendly Apricot Bar for a Morning Power Boost

When you are feeling lazy on a Monday morning, you just want to go back to bed. And a heavy breakfast will make you feel even heavier. But, an apricot bar won't. Just grab it on the go and you will feel energized for hours.

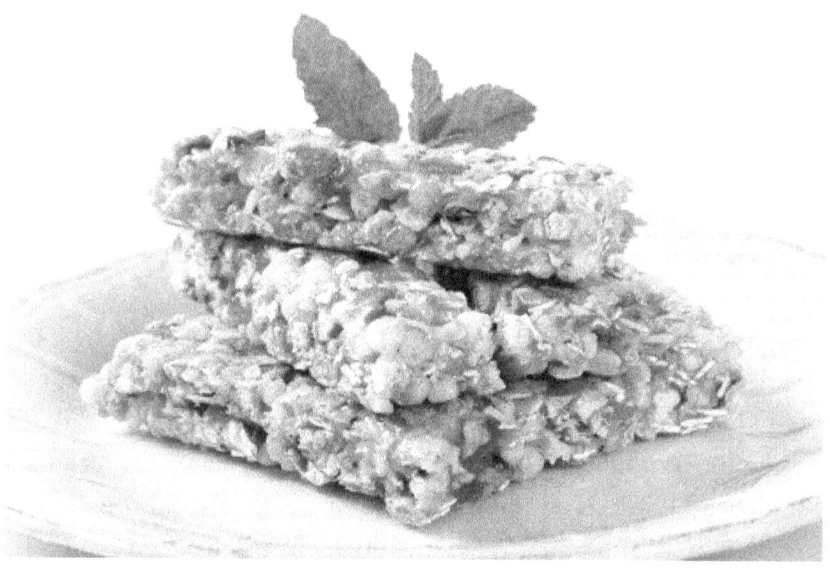

SERVES: 2
PREPARATION TIME: 15 min
INGREDIENTS:
Dried apricots 1 cup
Pecans 2 cups
Large eggs 2
Celtic sea salt 1 teaspoon
Vanilla extract 1 tablespoon
Chocolate chips ½ cup (optional)
METHOD:

1. Take a food processor and put pecans and apricots in it. Run the food processor and pulse until a coarse texture is

obtained.

2. Put in salt, vanilla and eggs and pulse until a ball of the mixture is formed.

3. Put the mixture in a baking dish, measuring approximately 8x8 inch.

4. Set the temperature of the oven at 350 degrees and bake the mixture for 25 minutes.

5. Let it cool and cut it into 3x3 inches square pieces. Serve.

Casserole For a Healthy Heart

This deliciously baked casserole is ideal for a healthy and quick breakfast. The goodness of vegetables and the flavor of breakfast sausage is all you need for a sumptuous breakfast.

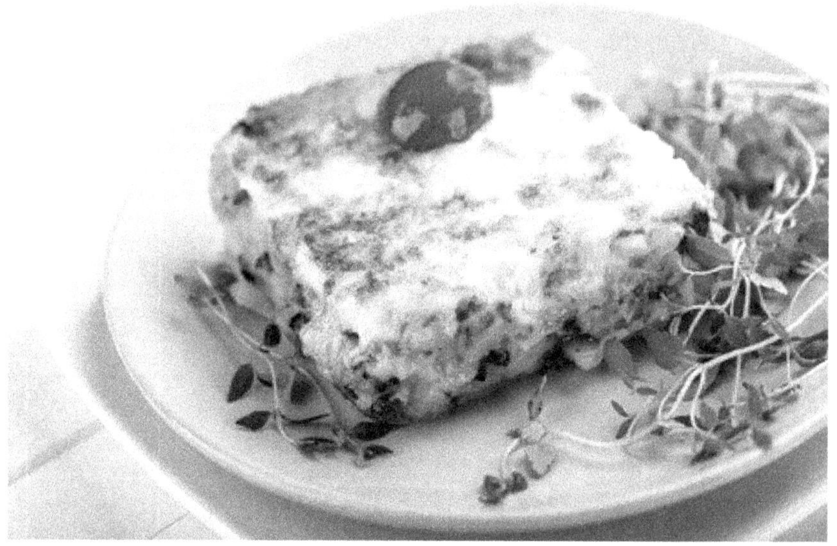

SERVES: 8-10
PREPARATION TIME: 30 min
INGREDIENTS:
Sugar free pork breakfast sausage 1 pound
Large sweet potato 1
Chopped baby spinach 2-3 cups
Diced green onion 1
Large eggs 10-12
Sea salt as per taste
Freshly ground pepper as per taste
Coconut oil or grass-fed butter for greasing
METHOD:

1. Preheat your oven to 375 degrees. Take a baking dish, approximately 9x13 inches, and grease it with the coconut oil

or grass fed butter.

2. Chop the spinach and dice the potato and green onions. Keep them aside separately.

3. Take a skillet and heat it to medium or high. Put breakfast sausage into it. Cook it well until it gets brown. Take the sausage out from the skillet and let the grease of the sausage remain in the skillet.

4. Add diced potatoes to the skillet and cook for about 10-15 minutes or till they become tender. Take them out into a bowl after cooking.

5. Toss the sweet potatoes with green onion, spinach, sausage, pepper and salt. Combine them well.

6. Spread the mixture evenly in the baking dish.

7. Whisk eggs in a separate bowl and pour the whisked eggs over the mixture in the baking dish.

8. Bake the mixture in the preheated oven until set or for 25-30 minutes.

9. Let it cool slightly. Cut it into square pieces and serve.

A Quick Breakfast with a Frozen Waffle

Let go back to the dinosaur age once again, but with a twist. These waffles are made with all the ancient ingredients but modern techniques. We know that you love to gobble down your food like a kid. And we are sure you will do the same with these waffles.

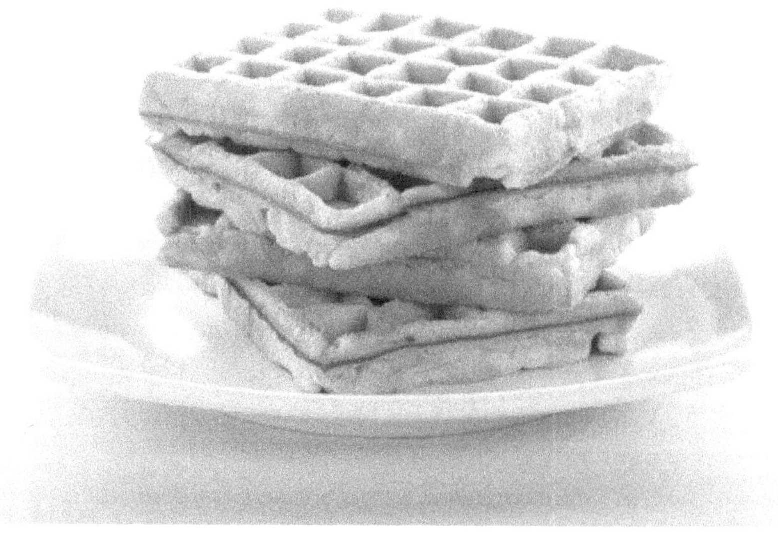

SERVES: 2
PREPARATION TIME: 15 min
INGREDIENTS:
Medium banana 1
Cored and peeled medium apple 1
Almond butter 1 cup or 8 ounces
Medium eggs 2
Arrowroot powder 1 tablespoon
Vanilla extract 1 tablespoon
Baking soda ½ teaspoon
Coconut oil 1 tablespoon (for greasing)
METHOD:

1. Make a puree of banana and apple in the food processor.

2. Attach a whisk attachment on the mixer. Whip the almond butter until fluffy and smooth, for 2-3 minutes.
3. Add all the ingredients and the puree to the almond butter. Whip all the ingredients to combine them.
4. Heat the waffle maker and grease it. Grease it every time for each waffle.
5. Take about 1 ladle of the batter for an 8x4 inch waffle. Put it into the waffle maker and cook for 3-5 minutes or until browned. Do not fill the waffle maker completely. Leave 40% space empty for the batter to spread.
6. If you feel that the waffle is soft, cook it for an extra minute.
7. You can serve it right away or store them flat in a freezer. Reheat them before eating again.

Benefits of Nuts and Coconut in the Porridge

Healthy nuts with this recipe will keep you full for quite a while. When you have a craving for a nourishing and warm breakfast, this porridge is the absolute hit in the Paleo diet plan. You will find that it is not very chewy, but it is a delicious substitute.

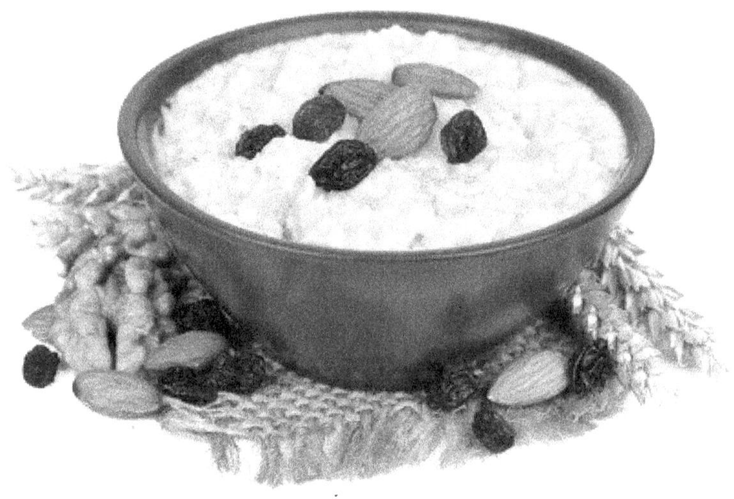

SERVES: 1
PREPARATION TIME: 10 min
INGREDIENTS:
Coconut flour 3 tablespoons
Coconut (finely shredded) 2 tablespoons
Coconut milk (canned) 1 cup
Water ¼ cup
Pasteurized egg 1 or ½ banana if you want an eggless option
Nuts toppings according to choice
METHOD:

1. Take a saucepan. Put coconut milk, shredded coconut and coconut flour into the saucepan over medium heat.

2. Mix the ingredients well and bring them to boil. When it thickens, lower the heat and cover the saucepan with a lid. Cook for 3 minutes. Stir in between.
3. Take off the saucepan and crack the egg into it. Whisk the egg quickly so that it does not get scrambled with the heat.
4. Place the saucepan over the heat again and cook for 2 more minutes.
5. If you want an eggless porridge, follow the same procedure. But, instead of adding egg, whisk in the mashed banana.
6. Serve with your favorite toppings.

Stir-Fried Power Punch Bacon

Bored with having eggs for breakfast? You are going to love this bacon recipe. This tasty bacon breakfast will give you a much needed kick start for a wonderful day. The lutein and vitamin C in bacon is very healthy for the eyes. You can also control your blood sugar with this delicious breakfast.

SERVES: 2

PREPARATION TIME: 20 min

INGREDIENTS:

Diced bacon slices 7-8

Yellow onion (diced) half

Potato (diced) 1

Zucchini (diced) 1

Beans 7

Avocado 1

Freshly ground black pepper as per taste

METHOD:

1. Take a medium sized skillet and cook the diced bacon over medium heat till the fat is drained. Take out the bacon and place in a bowl.
2. Take a sauté pan and heat it over medium heat.
3. Take out 1 tablespoon bacon fat from the skillet and put it into the sauté pan.
4. Put sweet potato and onion into the sauté pan. Cook until the onions and potato become tender. It may take 12-15 minutes.
5. Add diced zucchini and the beans to the mixture. Cook for 2 minutes.
6. Combine the bacon with the vegetables.
7. Put some freshly ground pepper and stir. Add sea salt if you wish. Serve hot.

Paleo Coconut Curry

This is one recipe you cannot go wrong with. There are so many interesting ingredients like ginger, garlic and basil. When you combine the beautiful ingredients of this recipe even in more or less proportion, you do not have to worry. You will not mess it up. At last, you will definitely make something delicious. It is an amazing treat for lunch with your family.

If you want to make a quick lunch, you can speed up the process. Use 2 frying pans-one for cooking the potatoes and the other for preparing the remaining ingredients. Plus, you would also need a spiralizer for making noodles of sweet potato. Smallest blade of the spiralizer is best.

Just go ahead and quickly cook it. Your kids must be screaming for lunch!

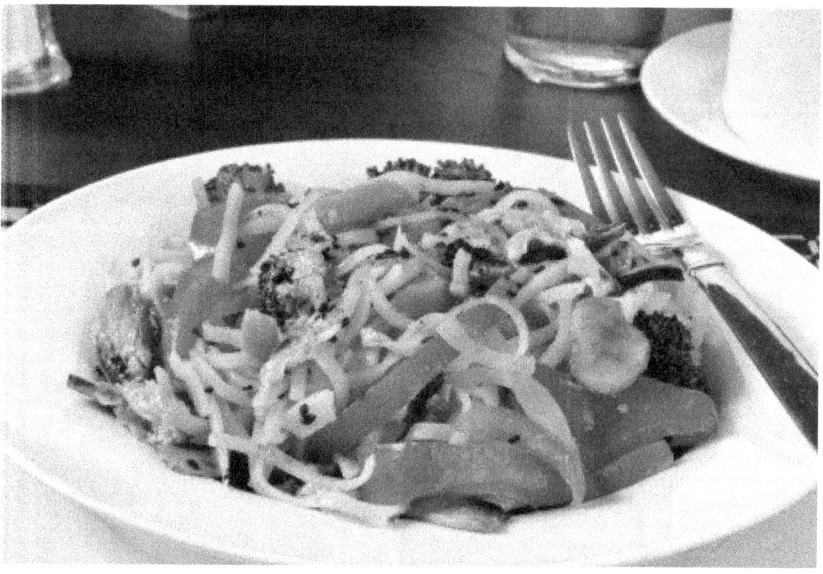

PREPARATION TIME: 30 min
INGREDIENTS:
Coconut oil 1 tablespoon
Chicken thighs 3-4 (chopped)
Sliced onion 1 small

Chopped red pepper 1
Salt as per taste
Pepper as per taste
SAUCE:
Coconut oil 1 tablespoon
Minced garlic cloves 2-3
Freshly grated ginger 2 teaspoons
Salt half or ¾ teaspoon
Curry powder 1 tablespoon
Heavy coconut cream 1 can
Starch (arrowroot, potato or tapioca) ½ teaspoon
Spiralized sweet potato 3
Lime juice 1 teaspoon
Cashews (optional)
METHOD:
<u>Step 1:</u>

1. For making sauce, put coconut oil in a pan and heat over low-medium heat.
2. Add minced garlic, chopped ginger, curry powder and salt. Cook for a few seconds.
3. Add coconut cream and mix well. You can also take any other cream if you want.
4. Lower the heat and add starch. The sauce will begin to thicken gradually.
5. Add spiralized potato to the sauce when the sauce is ready.

<u>Step 2:</u>

1. Season the chopped chicken thighs with pepper and salt. The chicken should be chopped into Small bite-sized pieces.
2. Take a separate pan while the potato cooks. Add coconut oil (1 tablespoon) to this pan and heat over medium low heat.

3. Add chicken and cook it well.
4. Add the sliced onions and cook for a few seconds.
5. Add pepper and cook for 2 minutes.
6. Put the chicken into the other pan of sauce. Pour in lime juice and stir well.
7. The coconut chicken curry is ready. Serve hot.

Paleo Gluten Free Lunch Recipes

Lunch is the most awaited meal at schools as well as in offices. Since breakfast is normally light on the diet chart, having a sumptuous lunch attains even more importance. Still, some people complain that they cannot "waste" time on a lunch break. Their claim of being too busy takes its toll on them in the long term. Lunch skippers either work during the lunch break or they meet with the HR department to discuss their performance. How can your performance improve when all you do is work? Even your computer needs a break. When a machine cannot function without rest, how can you?

Benefits of lunch

Of course you know that you need food to live. But, what kind of food? Have you felt that your regular lunch makes you feel drowsy and that is why you do not feel like having it? Or you might give lame excuse about being too busy to have lunch. Well, the Paleo diet will fade away all your excuses.

Research has found out that taking a lunch break, even if it is short, improves your overall performance throughout the rest of the day and your decision-making process as well. When we are at the workplace, we need to manage a lot of things. We need to have self control over emotions, thoughts, behavior and urges. Besides adequate sleep and regular vacations, our meals have a very important role to play in our resource recovery. Experts say that people have a better thought process and concentration to process information given to them after lunch.

Having a good lunch break also fights fatigue throughout the day. We can give you a thousand more benefits of having a satisfactory lunch break. But, the best way is to observe it yourself.

Here, we are listing a few Paleo lunch recipes for you which will keep you even more energized than the regular grainy lunch. The previous meals you had might have made you feel sleepy after lunch. It is a common practice among office workers to keep their stomach half empty just to stay "awake" at the office and "survive" the afternoon.

But, now you do not have to worry so much if you have a Paleo lunch. The recipes are proven to keep you awake and active for the rest of the day. So let us start with the Paleo lunch.

The Nutrients of Cilantro Packed in Baked Lime Chicken

After reading the vegan recipes of the breakfast section, you might have been missing some meat. So here is the one recipe you were looking for. The yummy flavors of cilantro and lime in the chicken breast are mouthwatering. Baking the chicken gives the flavors a chance to infuse through the dish. You can also grill it if you prefer it like that. Lunch could not be healthier and tastier!

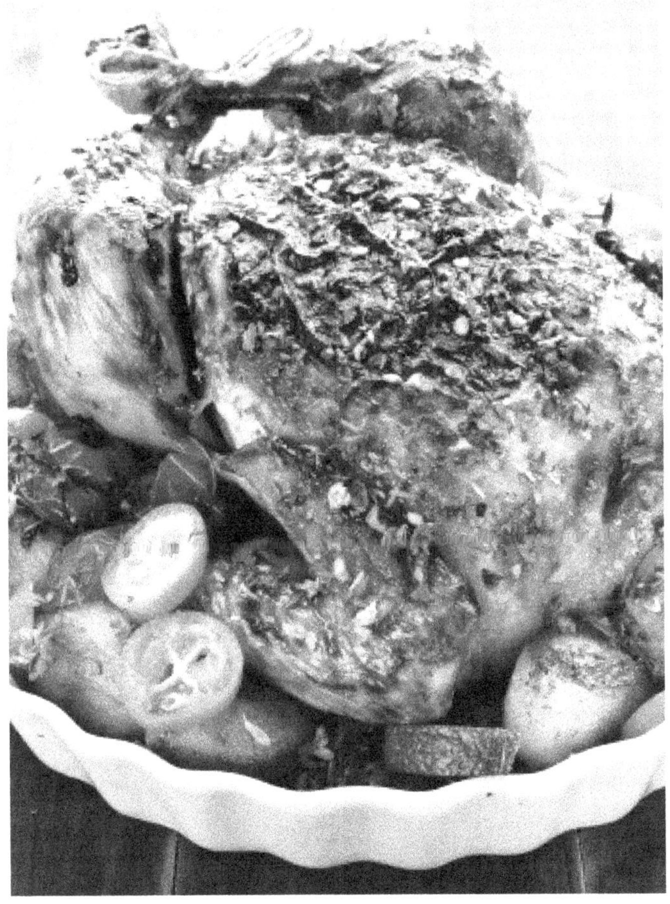

SERVES: 2

PREPARATION TIME: 30 minutes for cooking, 4-6 hours for marinating.

INGREDIENTS:

Chicken breast (boneless and skinless) 1 pound
Fresh lime juice ½ cup
Chopped fresh cilantro ½ cup
Dijon mustard ¼ cup
Olive oil 1 tablespoon
Chilli powder 1 tablespoon
Celtic sea salt ½ teaspoon
Pepper ½ teaspoon

METHOD:

1. Put cilantro, lime juice, olive oil, mustard, chilli powder, pepper and salt in a food processor and run to combine the ingredients well.
2. Rinse the boneless chicken breasts. Pat them dry.
3. Place them in a baking dish, approx. 7x11 inches.
4. Pour the mixture from the food processor over the chicken breasts. Cover the dish and marinate it for 4-6 hours. If you are in a hurry, give it at least half an hour.
5. Preheat the oven at 350 degrees. Put in the baking dish and cook for 22 minutes.
6. Take out and pour any extra sauce if you like.
7. Serve hot.

<u>The Tangy Flavor of Spices in a Tomato and Tuna Burger</u>

What else can be better for lunch than tuna when it is cheap, healthy and full of protein? The recipe mentioned below is so versatile that you can eat with some salad, or stir it together with some rice, mix it through pasta or just simply make a burger out of it. Whatever you do, the flavor is going to be awesome. Go to your backyard and grab the natural ingredients mentioned below.

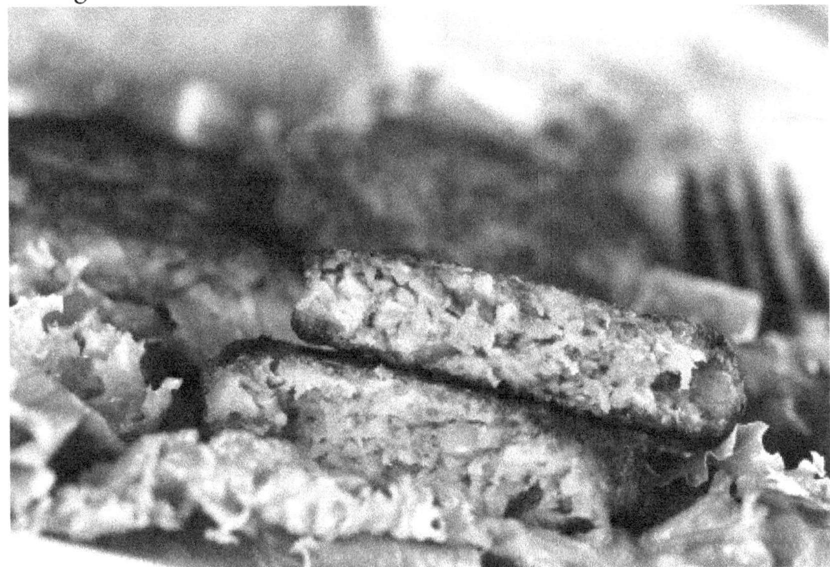

SERVES: 1
PREPARATION TIME: 25 minutes
INGREDIENTS:
Tuna 1 cup (4 cans of tuna drained, rinsed)
Chopped Spanish onion 1
Small chopped red chilli 1
Crushed garlic clove 1
Egg 1
Tomato paste 2 tablespoons
Coconut flour 1 tablespoon
Salt as per taste

Pepper as per taste
SERVING (optional):
Sliced Avocado
Lettuce
Onion rings
Extra chilli
Fresh coriander (cilantro)
METHOD:

1. Preheat the oven to 175 degrees.
2. Line a baking tray using parchment paper or baking paper.
3. Put onion, red chilli, tuna, egg, garlic, tomato paste, coconut flour, salt and pepper into a bowl and combine them properly.
4. Divide the mixture into 6 and flatten into 6 evenly sized burger patties.
5. Place the patties on the baking tray.
6. Place the tray into the oven and cook for 10 minutes.
7. While the burgers are cooking, take a serving bowl and place 2 lettuce leaves on it. Top with some sliced avocado. You can also use some cream or yoghurt if you are not a strict Paleo.
8. Sprinkle some fresh cilantro, ringed onions and some chopped chilli.
9. Place the burgers over the serving ingredients. Serve hot.

Tasty Tostones for a Wholesome Meal

If you like to indulge in a lot of flavors with some tangy tastes and lots of ingredients, this recipe is the right one for you. The tasty tostones or nachos are made with a unique recipe for you to enjoy. It is easy to prepare and will completely satiate your taste buds. Indulge in the marvelous taste and you will want to have more every time.

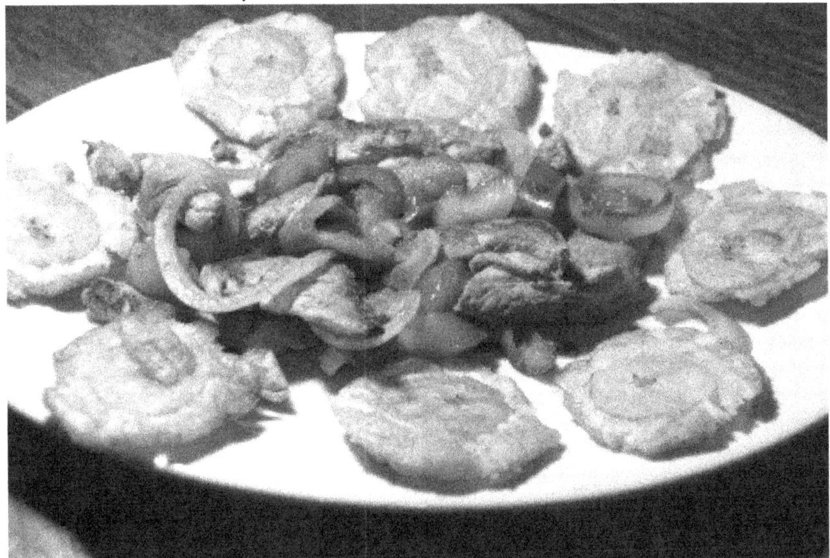

SERVES: 3

PREPARATION TIME: 30-40 minutes

INGREDIENTS:

Nachos or Tostones:

Coconut oil ¼ cup

Plantains or bananas (ripe and yellow) 2

Beef:

Ground beef 140 grams

Chopped onion 1

Minced garlic 4 cloves

Coconut oil 2 teaspoons

Sea salt ¼ teaspoon

Guacamole or avocado dip:

Avocado ½

Small onion ¼

Garlic powder ¼ teaspoon

Lime juice (optional) 1 teaspoon

Sea salt 1/8 teaspoon

<u>Sour cream:</u>

Coconut cream ¼ cup

Lemon juice 2 teaspoons

Raw honey 2 teaspoons

Sea salt only a pinch

METHOD:

<u>First fry:</u>

1. Cut the plantains or bananas into slices about ½ inch thick.
2. Take a large shallow frying pan and pour ¼ cup coconut oil in it. Heat the oil over a medium flame and fry the bananas for about 3 minutes.
3. Flip them over and fry for 3 minutes again on the other side.
4. When the bananas turn yellow, you can take them out.
5. Let them cool on a wire rack.

<u>Second fry:</u>

1. When you find that the bananas are cool enough that you can handle them, you need to flatten them. You do not have to mash them. Just flatten them.
2. Toss the flattened bananas in the same fry pan and fry them for the second time. Add some more oil if you feel the need to.
3. Fry them until golden brown.
4. Take them out and place them on the wire rack. Season them with salt.

Cooking the meat:

1. Heat coconut oil in a frying pan and put onions and garlic into it. Sauté over medium heat.
2. When the onions turn brown, add beef and fry. Stir at intervals until you see that there are no pink spots.
3. Leave the meat to turn brown for 2 minutes on low-medium heat. Keep it aside.

Guacamole or avocado dip:
Combine all the ingredients in a food processor.

Sour cream
Combine all the ingredients in a food processor.

Serve:
Place the bananas on a round plate. Layer the beef mixture over the plantains or bananas. Spread some avocado dip or guacamole over the beef. Pour some sour cream over the beef. When the ingredients are loaded in the plate, serve.

Enjoy the beef with each bite of plantain.

Joyful Jalapeno Burgers with Chicken

The amazing flavor of chicken and jalapeno along with Asian ingredients makes this burger a standalone contender in this Paleo cookbook. You can gobble it down alone or with guacamole. You are going to love this smooth burger anyhow.

You can make some variations with the chicken if you want. You can use beef or turkey as well. Grill it carefully and your family is going to love it forever.

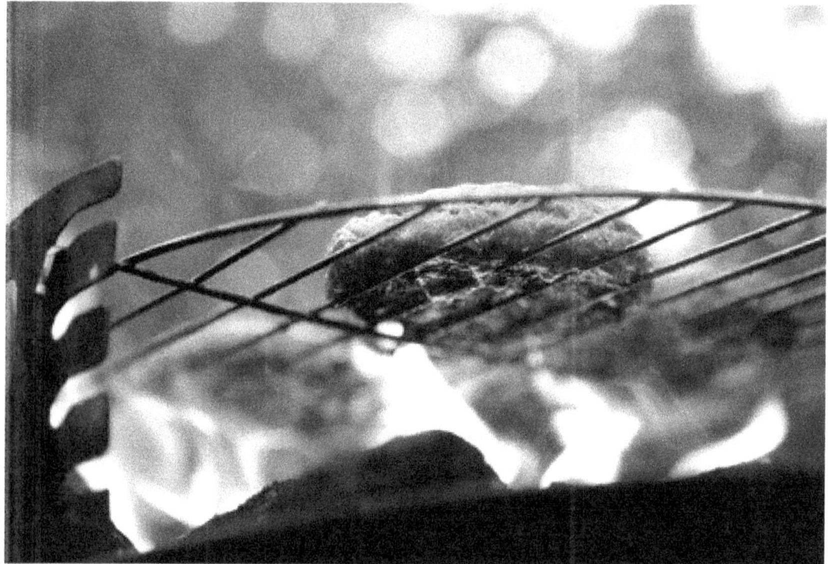

SERVES: 4
PREPARATION TIME: 25 min
INGREDIENTS:
<u>Burger patties:</u>
Ground chicken 1.5 pounds
Diced white onion 2/3 cup
Chopped fresh cilantro or coriander ¼ cup
Minced garlic cloves 2 teaspoons
Seeded and diced jalapeno 2 teaspoons
Cumin 1 teaspoon

Paprika 1 teaspoon

Red pepper flakes 1 teaspoon

<u>Guacamole or avocado dip:</u>

Avocado ½

Small onion ¼

Garlic powder ¼ teaspoon

Lime juice (optional) 1 teaspoon

Sea salt 1/8 teaspoon

<u>Sour cream:</u>

Coconut cream ¼ cup

Lemon juice 2 teaspoons

Raw honey 2 teaspoons

Sea salt only a pinch

METHOD:

<u>Burger patties:</u>

1. Clean your hands and mix the following ingredients in a large bowl with your hands: ground chicken, cilantro, onion, garlic, ground cumin, jalapeño, red pepper flakes and paprika.
2. Divide the mixture into 4 equal parts and make burger patties.
3. Grill the patties over medium-low heat.
4. Flip over when the patty stops sticking to the grates of the grill.
5. Cook the other side until well cooked.

<u>Guacamole or avocado dip:</u>

You have made this before in the previous recipe. It tastes equally good with this burger patty as well.

You just have to combine all the ingredients in a food processor.

<u>Sour cream:</u>

Combine all the ingredients in a food processor.

<u>Serving directions:</u>

Prepare the guacamole and sour cream beforehand. Serve the burgers hot with these add-ons. You can also gobble them down alone if you want to.

<u>Storage directions:</u>

If you want to freeze them, do it without cooking them, using parchment paper. Freeze them in a freezer bag. On the day of serving, you can take them out and grill as per cooking directions.

Paleo Chicken Wraps

Wraps are one of the favorite lunch dishes in America. Besides the fact that they are easy to make, they taste amazing too. You can have them at your leisure or when you are in a hurry. Fill the wrap with your favorite stuffing and quickly wrap it up. It is such a quick food that even your 10-year-old-baby girl can also try her hand at it.

Here, we are going to make a delicious wrap minus the refined flour tortilla. We will use lettuce instead. Make sure you use an extra layer of lettuce than you think will be needed so that if one layer tears, the other one saves the stuffing from bursting out.

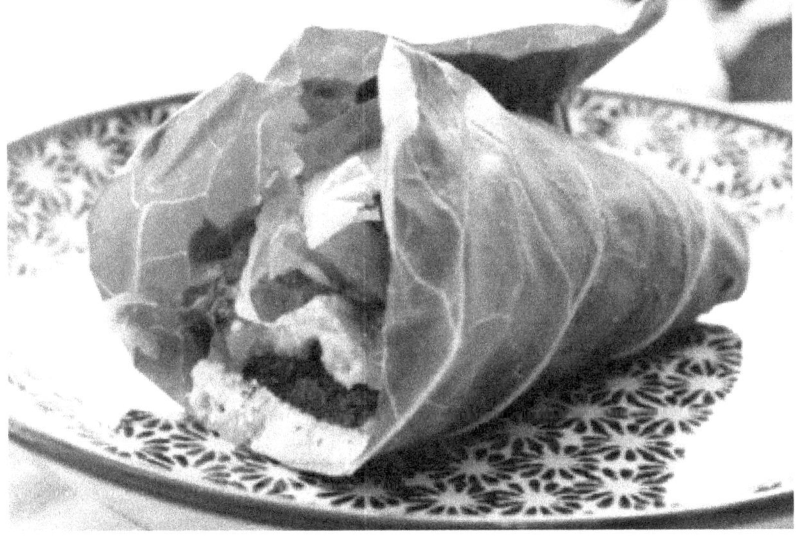

SERVES: 4

PREPARATION TIME: 25 min

INGREDIENTS:

Chicken breasts (skinless, boneless) 1 pound

Olive oil (extra virgin) 2 tablespoons

Sliced tomato 1 medium

Chopped avocado 1

Cooked and crumbled bacon 6 strips

Homemade Paleo mayonnaise 4 tablespoon

(Refer to next recipe for homemade Paleo mayonnaise)
Butter lettuce leaves/ Iceberg lettuce 8 large
Paprika ½ teaspoon
Cooking fat
Sea salt as per taste
Freshly ground pepper as per taste
METHOD:

1. Preheat a skillet or grill to medium or high heat.
2. Season the boneless and skinless chicken on both sides with sea salt, paprika, and black pepper.
3. Grill the chicken on a grill or cook in a skillet using cooking fat.
4. Flip over when it is cooked on one side. Cook until there is no pink visible.
5. Keep it aside for cooling for 5 minutes.
6. Break the chicken into small bite-sized pieces.

<u>**To make wraps:**</u>

1. Take two lettuce leaves and spread them with some mayonnaise. Top them with bacon, chicken, tomato and avocado.
2. Roll the lettuce leaves and secure them in place using a toothpick or kitchen dart.
3. Cut the wraps in half before serving.

Homemade Paleo Mayonnaise

If you thought that you would never be able to devour mayonnaise because you turned Paleo, here is good news for you. We have brought you a delicious recipe for homemade Paleo mayonnaise. You won't have to shell out dollars for that expensive mayonnaise available in the supermarket. So, now you can indulge in your favorite burgers and chicken wraps with this purely Paleo mayonnaise. You have two options of mayo here: Baconnaise and the mayo made of coconut oil.

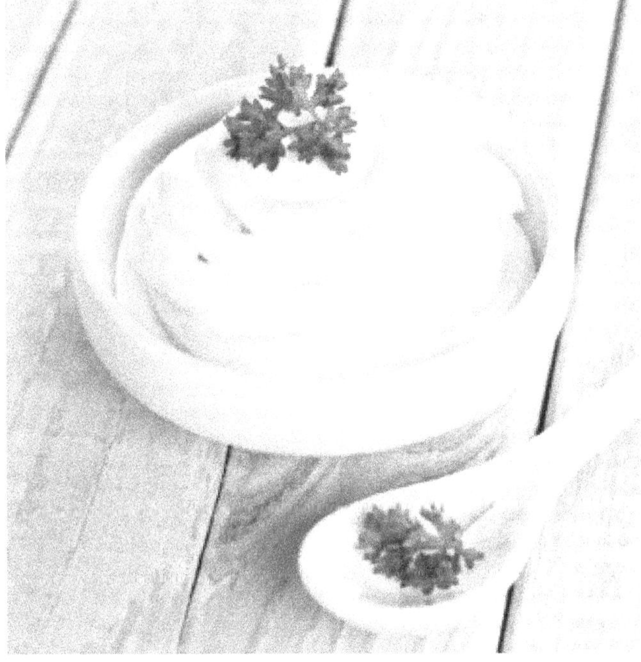

Coconut Oil Paleo Mayonnaise
YOU WILL MAKE: 1.25 cup
PREPARATION TIME: 15 min
INGREDIENTS:
Egg yolks 2
Mustard 1 teaspoon
Lemon juice 3 teaspoons
Olive oil ½ cup

Coconut oil ` ½ cup
<u>Baconnaise:</u>
Bacon fat 1 cup
(In place of olive oil and coconut oil)
METHOD:

1. Mix mustard, egg yolks and lemon juice (1 teaspoon) in a bowl or blender.
2. Drip oil drop by drop into the mixture and blend at the lowest speed. Do not hurry it too much. Pour more oil in only when the earlier ingredients are mixed properly. Else, the oil will separate and it will become difficult to handle.
3. As you keep adding oil, the mayonnaise will become thick. You can add larger amounts of oil at this point.
4. When you have blended in all the olive oil and coconut oil, pour in the remaining lemon juice and blend.
5. Add pepper and salt.
6. Serve as it is or cold, as you like it. Indulge without guilt.

(Use bacon fat in place of oils if you want to make Baconnaise)

Paleo Gluten Free Dinner Recipes

So after you have read about the importance of breakfast and lunch, you must be thinking now I am here again to bore you with the benefits of dinner. But, I cannot resist telling you a few pleasing facts about a Paleo dinner.

The whole world talks about the kick-start to the day that a healthy breakfast gives, and the re-fueling of the body that happens through a sumptuous lunch. But, there are hardly any debates on the quality and timing of dinner. Even Paleo followers tend to have a non-Paleo dinner because they are tired of having a Paleo diet throughout the day.

Here, we will talk in brief about the importance of a healthy and timely dinner.

When should you have dinner?

Say goodbye to late night meals and try to have your dinner around 7pm-8pm. This will not only keep you healthy but also give you a slimmer waist. Resist the temptation of eating late at night. Instead, you can sleep early and wake up earlier. Nobody feels hungry when they're sleeping! Do this for a week and you will definitely feel better. You should also avoid taking heavy meals at night. Loads of food at night takes longer to digest and hence you might face problems in having a deep sleep.

Owing to the modern lifestyle, avoiding late night parties and dinners is not always possible. Thus, you can do one thing to maintain your biological cycle. Have some light Paleo snacks after sunset. Do not stay hungry to eat at the party. In fact, when you eat early, you will not feel hungry late at night. Thus, your health can remain as good as you want it to be.

What should you have for dinner?

When you reach your fridge at dinner time, sometimes you feel that the fridge is exploding with options. At other times, you might feel that you just need an escape route to come out of the daily dilemma of cooking and just order from the local restaurant. But, just because you are on a slimming regime does not mean that you have to survive on a skimpy salad bowl.

The Paleo diet recipes we have mentioned in the following chapters will make you take wise decisions daily to cook a sumptuous and healthy dinner for your family. You can have the food in generous amounts but at a good time as I have already mentioned above. Feel free to savour the delicious Paleo recipes and still get a good night's sleep.

A Great Gravy for Paleo Lovers

Every day is a day of dilemma for busy moms, who wonder at 5pm, what to cook for dinner? Here, we have listed a delicious gravy recipe for you. Since you are on a Paleo diet, you might feel sometimes that the main course is incomplete. You can compliment any burger, grilled chicken or nachos with this gravy. You can even serve it as a soup.

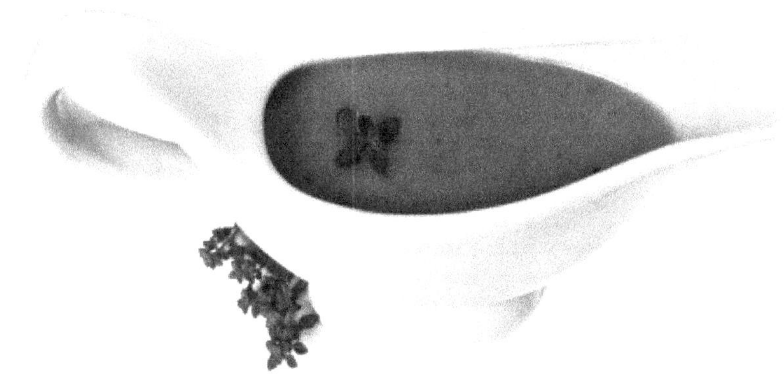

SERVES: 4
PREPARATION TIME: 25-30 min
INGREDIENTS:
Green-fed butter 2 tablespoons
Finely chopped onion 1
Black pepper ¼ teaspoon
Starch from arrowroot, potato or tapioca 1.5 tablespoons
Almond flour (blanched) 5-6 tablespoon
Chicken broth 1.25 cup
Garlic powder 1/2 teaspoon
Heavy cream/ coconut milk (heavy) 1 tablespoon (optional)
Salt as per taste

METHOD:

1. Preheat a saucepan and add onion and butter. Cook for 20 minutes over low medium heat or until the onions are brown.
2. Add almond flour, starch and black pepper. Stir continuously for a minute.
3. Add rest of the ingredients.
4. Stir at intervals until the gravy is thickened.
5. If you want to make it thicker, you can add 2-3 tablespoons of almond flour.
6. Add salt as per taste.
7. Let it cool for a while.
8. You can pulse it in a food processor to grind the onions and attain a smooth texture. But this is completely up to you. If you like it as it is, just go ahead and serve.
9. The gravy will thicken even more as it settles.

Frittata to Freshen You Up

Now we come to a recipe which does not need many ingredients from the market. You can put in whatever you have in your refrigerator and a Paleo delicacy is ready. Have it for breakfast, lunch or dinner, this frittata with sausage will energize you.

If you like to experiment with the given recipes, just make sure whatever you include in the recipe, is packed with flavor.

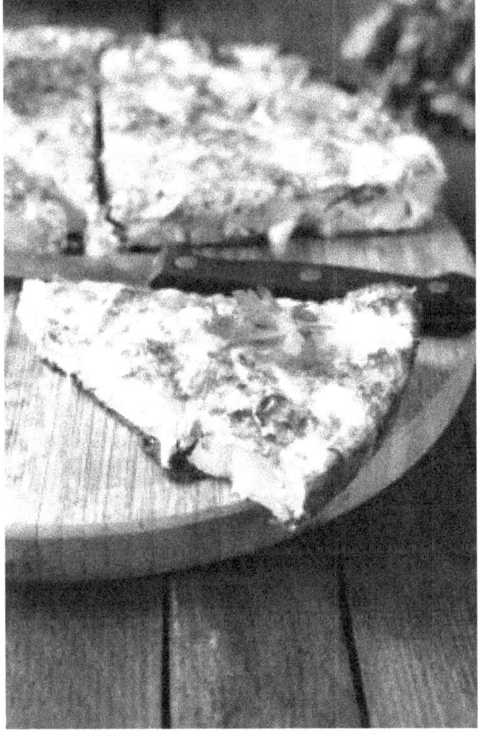

SERVES: 3-4
PREPARATION TIME: 30-40 min
INGREDIENTS:

Sausage:

Ground pork 1 pound
Rubbed sage 1 teaspoon
Sweet paprika (smoked) ½ teaspoon

Hot paprika (smoked) ½ teaspoon

Sea salt 1 teaspoon

Freshly ground pepper ¾ teaspoon

<u>Frittata:</u>

Bacon fat 1 tablespoon

Sausage (crumbled and chopped) 3 ounces

Diced onion ¼ cup

Diced red pepper ¼ cup

Roasted and cubed butternut squash ½ cup

Eggs 3 (large)

Fresh herbs (mixed) 2 teaspoons/ or dried herbs (1/2 teaspoon)

Sea salt as per taste

Pepper as per taste

METHOD:

<u>For sausages:</u>

1. Mix all the spices in a large bowl.
2. Add them to the ground pork. Combine them well.
3. Divide the mixture into 8 equal portions and make patties.
4. Cook the patties in a skillet in extra virgin olive oil.
5. Cook well until they are brown.

<u>For frittata:</u>

1. Preheat your oven.
2. Beat the eggs, pepper, herbs and salt until they are combined well.
3. Pour the bacon fat into an ovenproof skillet.
4. Sauté onions with pepper until soft.
5. Add sausages, squash them and cook well.
6. Pour the egg mixture into the skillet and cook until the edges begin to set.
7. Put the skillet in the oven.

8. Broil it until you see the frittata gets brown and puffed. It takes approximately 3-5 minutes.
9. Serve hot.

Piccata with Chunky Chicken

Here we are again with another delicious chicken recipe. The amazing blend of flavors in this chicken with sauce is just heavenly. The capers earn the brownie points in taste. This is a satisfying, filling dish for dinner. Just forget everything else and devour this gratifying dish.

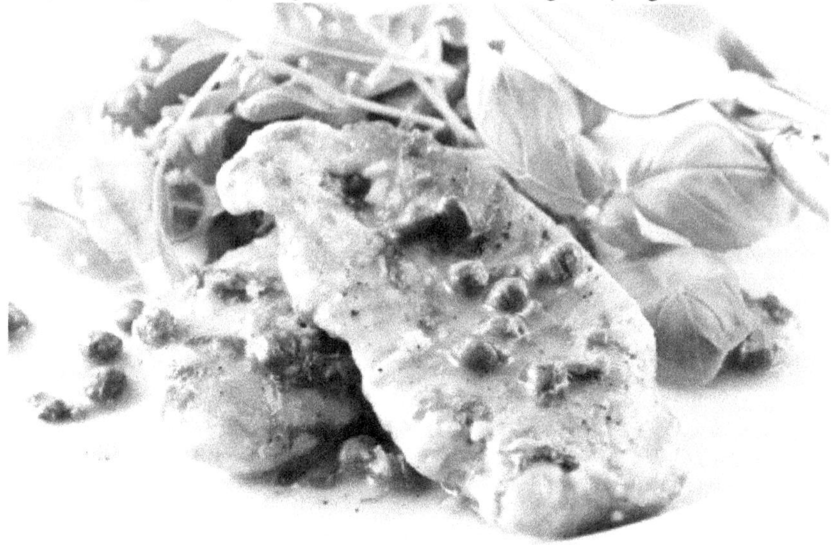

SERVES: 3-4
PREPARATION TIME: 30-40 min
INGREDIENTS:
Chicken breasts (skinless, boneless) 1.5 pounds
Almond flour (blanched) ½ cup
Sea salt (Celtic) ½ teaspoon
Spices and herbs mix (readymade) ½ teaspoon
Grapeseed oil 5 tablespoons
Olive oil 5 tablespoons
Lemon juice ¼ cup
Chicken stock 1 cup
Brined capers ¼ cup
Freshly chopped parsley ¼ cup

METHOD:

1. Place the chicken breasts horizontally and cut them into half. If the chicken breasts are too large, cut them into two pieces each after you have halved them.
2. Put the chicken between two sheets of parchment paper.
3. Beat them with a heavy object such as a skillet, until they are ¼ inch thick.
4. Combine the herb mix, salt and almond flour.
5. Rinse the chicken in water and toss them through the mixture of almond flour.
6. Take them out when they are coated with the flour mixture.
7. Put grape seed oil (2 tablespoons) and olive oil in a skillet and heat on a medium to high heat.
8. Put 3-4 chicken pieces into the skillet and cook for 3 minutes on each side or until brown.
9. Repeat the cooking process with all the pieces of chicken and take them out onto a plate.
10. Keep warm the plate in a preheated oven.
11. Add capers, chicken stock and lemon juice to the skillet. Soften the browned bits with a metal spatula so that they get incorporated into the sauce.
12. Cook the sauce until it is reduced by half. Pour in the remaining grape seed oil (3 tablespoons) and whisk.
13. Take the chicken from the oven, and pour some sauce over it. You can also sprinkle on some parsley before serving.

Chicken with Honey Glaze

Delicious chicken glazed with honey tastes as delicious as it looks. The sesame seeds to coat the chicken are tasty plus they are healthy too. Serve it with the sriracha sauce and your family is going to kiss your hands for cooking such a beautiful dinner!

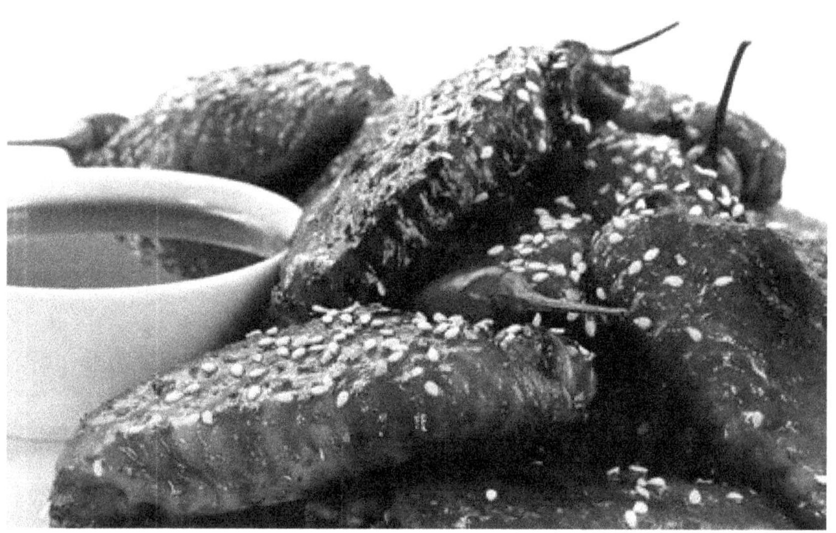

SERVES: 3-4

PREPARATION TIME: 50 min

INGREDIENTS:

Chicken:

Chicken breast 1 pound

Chinese five spice 2 teaspoons

Cayenne pepper ¼ teaspoon

Sea salt 1 teaspoon

Freshly ground black pepper ¼ teaspoon

Organic honey 1 tablespoon

Lime juice 1 tablespoon

Sesame seeds 1 tablespoon

Chopped cilantro 3 tablespoons

Lime wedges 2 tablespoons

Sliced fresh chilli as per taste

<u>Sriracha:</u>

Jalapeno peppers (seeded, stemmed and chopped) 1.5 pound

Peeled and minced garlic 3 cloves

Vinegar (white wine) 1/3 cup

Tomato paste 3 tablespoons

Organic honey 3 tablespoons

Fish sauce 2 tablespoons

Sea salt 1.5 teaspoons

<u>Mayonnaise mixture:</u>

Homemade Paleo mayonnaise (recipe given) 3 tablespoons

Greek yoghurt 3 tablespoons

Lemon juice 1 teaspoon

Freshly ground black pepper as per taste

METHOD:

<u>Sriracha:</u>

1. Put all the ingredients into a blender and pulse until it becomes a smooth puree.
2. Pour the blended mixture into a saucepan.
3. Bring the mixture to boil at medium to high heat.
4. When it comes to boil, simmer the heat and cook for half an hour. Stir at frequent intervals.
5. Pour the sauce into a medium-sized jar and let it cool.
6. Refrigerate for storage.

<u>Sriracha Mayonnaise Mixture</u>

1. Take a bowl and mix Greek yoghurt, sriracha, mayonnaise, lime juice, pepper and stir well to combine.

2. Taste it and add more seasoning if needed.

<u>Chicken:</u>

1. Cut the chicken breasts into strips.
2. Mix cayenne pepper, five-spice, pepper and salt in a small bowl. Spread the mixture over a parchment paper sheet.
3. Coat the chicken with this spice mixture.
4. Fold over the parchment paper and slightly flatten the chicken using a rolling pin.
5. Mix honey, lime juice and olive oil in a small bowl.
6. Put the chicken into a large bag (ziplock) and pour the honey marinade mixture.
7. Marinate chicken for at least 30 minutes or 6 hours for maximum flavor.
8. After the marinating is done, heat a grill pan at medium high.
9. Cook the chicken for 4-5 minutes at each side.
10. Toss the chicken in some sesame seeds to coat well.
11. To serve, arrange the chicken on a serving platter with some lime wedges, and freshly sliced chilli. Sprinkle with cilantro.
12. Serve with some sriracha mayonnaise.

Zucchini Zoom Zoodles

Is it possible to eat pasta when you are on a Paleo diet? Sounds strange, right? It is possible! We will show you a recipe for zucchini noodles. They are also called zoodles. Wow! You can still have spaghetti with meatballs.

There are two easy methods for making zoodles. Firstly, you can use a julienne peeler to make noodles out of zucchini. Do not forget to remove the stem off the zucchini first.

Secondly, you can make zoodles with the same method listed above and then sauté them in a saucepan using olive oil.

We will use the second method for this recipe. These are healthier than traditional pasta, and tasty too. You can also use a spiralizer to make zucchini noodles, if you have one.

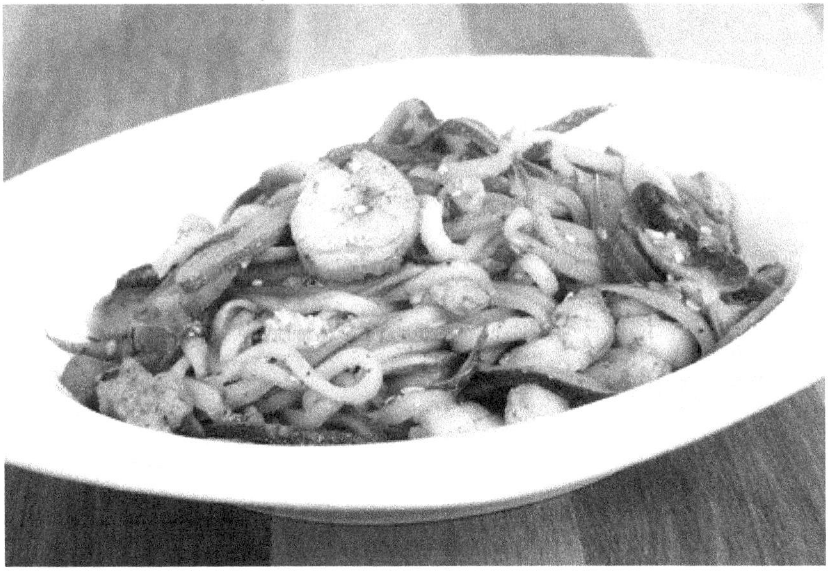

SERVES: 3-4
PREPARATION TIME: 30 min
INGREDIENTS:
Seasoning:

The fresh vegetables and herbs mentioned in the seasoning have to be dried and ground first. Then you can mix them in the spices.

Alternatively, you can also buy a readymade chef's shake from the supermarket, which contains all these ingredients. They are easily available.

To make a homemade seasoning, create a mixture of the following ingredients: onion, black pepper, celery seeds, red pepper, basil, marjoram, garlic, orange peel, carrots, tomato, parsley, lemon oil, bay leaf, lemon juice powder, thyme, oregano, savory, citric acid, cumin, rosemary, mustard, coriander.

<u>Zoodles:</u>

Olive oil 1 tablespoon

Zucchini 1 pound

Seasoning 1 teaspoon

METHOD:

1. Take a large sauté pan and heat olive oil on a medium flame.
2. Add seasoning and zoodles to the pan.
3. Stir the zoodles until they become tender (3-5 minutes).
4. Serve them with meatballs.

Paleo Mushroom Caps

This is a perfect dish for a birthday party. This recipe is so easy to make and likewise so easy to handle that you can keep it on the center table at your kid's birthday party. The guests and the kids can help themselves and pick a taco or two while they enjoy the party. You can keep it for the starters or as a substitute for salad. However you do it, you, your family and your guests are going to love it.

And if someone says that he did not like it, then he must be allergic to mushrooms. You do not have to bother about it. Wink! Let's get started.

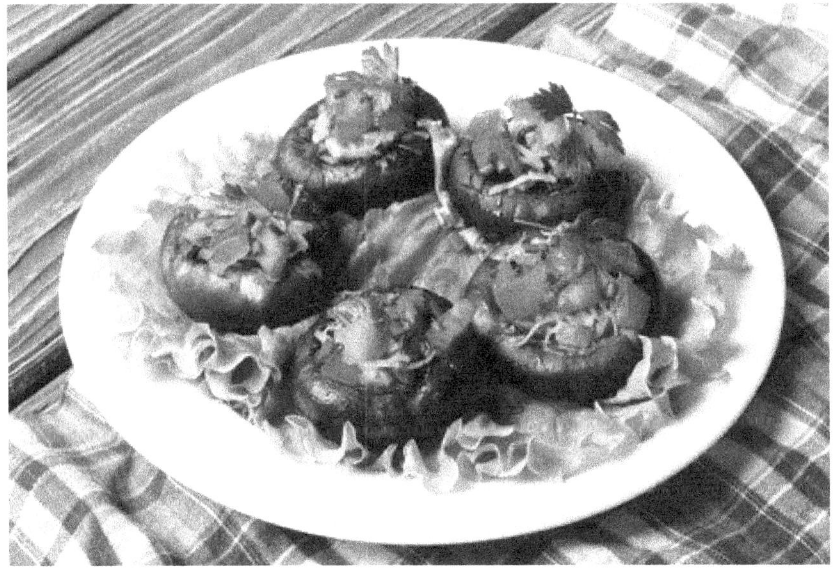

SERVES:
PREPARATION TIME:
INGREDIENTS:
Portobello mushrooms 4
Chopped onions ¼ large
Ground beef 0.7-1 pound
Diced red chilli 1
Garlic 1 clove

Clarified butter ½ tablespoon
Taco seasoning (Paleo) 2 tablespoon
Salt as per taste
TOPPINGS:
Cilantro ½ cup
Finely chopped green onions 2 medium
Sliced cherry tomatoes ½ cup
Sliced kalamata olives ½ cup
Guacamole ½ cup
METHOD:

1. Preheat your oven to 205 degrees Celsius.
2. Take a large frying pan and pour in the clarified butter.
3. Add onions and cook over medium heat.
4. Take out the stems of mushrooms while the onion cooks and dice them finely.
5. When the onions become soft, add the mushroom stems to the pan.
6. Add chilli pepper and ground beef and let it brown.
7. Add salt and taco seasoning.
8. Position the mushroom tacos in a baking dish and bake them for 10 minute (top down). Flip over after they are cooked from one side and then bake the other side for 10 minutes.
9. Fill up the baked mushrooms with the cooked beef. Top them with olives, green onions, tomatoes and finally with cilantro.
10. Serve it to your little kids.

Paleo Gluten Free Desserts

Finally, we are at the favorite part of our mealtime- the desserts. This is my favorite part too. You must be thinking what kind of desserts we can have in a Paleo diet, when we cannot include dairy products, breads, etc in our meals. But, I do have a solution for you. You will discover in the following chapter that the delicious desserts of the Paleo diet plan are actually made for freshening up your mood.

Being purely Paleo, we also do not recommend deviating from the wise path you have chosen. But, what should we do with our cravings that occur every week? We know that sometimes you really feel like eating something sweet and you cannot help it. Therefore, here we are, with some delicious purely Paleo desserts.

You do not need to have any guilt factor while having these desserts. I will tell you why:

How desserts can be healthy?

Paleo does not eliminate carbohydrate from your meals. Your body needs a limited amount of carbohydrates to maintain the nutrition level. The desserts mentioned in the coming chapters are custom-made to give you a restricted but ample supply of carbohydrates. They actually fuel your mind and body.

You must have jumped at the thought of having a chocolate pie. Haven't you? It is not just psychological, but physical too. Desserts are proven to lift up your mood. The nutrients in desserts boost the supply of happy hormones in your body which make you joyful while you eat your dessert.

Good news! Paleo desserts can help you lose and maintain your weight as well. Yes, that's correct! Whenever you have a craving of your sweet tooth, do not suppress it. When you eat desserts while maintaining your rest of the diet, you 'can' control your weight rather than completely eliminating sweets from your diet.

Combine your desserts with lots of fruits and you can be healthy as well as happy while you indulge in the "crime". Americans are already known to have less fruits than required. So you can compensate your fruit diet by combining as many fruits as possible in your sweets.

<u>Paleo desserts</u>

Now you have a number of beautiful healthy Paleo dessert options. Allow your sweet tooth a day off and gobble down these delicacies guilt free. But, how do you decide what kind of ingredients to put in your Paleo desserts? Don't worry. We are here to help you. Just go through the soothing sweets mentioned in the coming chapters. Once you get the hang of it, you can experiment with your own dessert recipes. Let us continue.

<u>Paleo Vanilla Coconut Ice-Cream</u>

Being a Paleo follower, you might not get everything ready-to-eat in the supermarkets, but there are ingredients available in abundance. These raw materials can be utilized in various forms to make something as tasty as a non-Paleo food.

Here, we are giving you a recipe for a Paleo ice-cream, which you would have thought that you cannot eat anymore. Ice-creams just need a little effort from you to make it of the same quality that you see in the market.

You do not need to buy an expensive ice-cream machine. Here is a simple trick to make a professional ice-cream. Cool the custard in a bowl in the fridge before you freeze it in the freezer. Whisk the custard every half an hour for 2-3 hours when freezing it. Putting in just this much effort will give you the same results that you'd get from a machine.

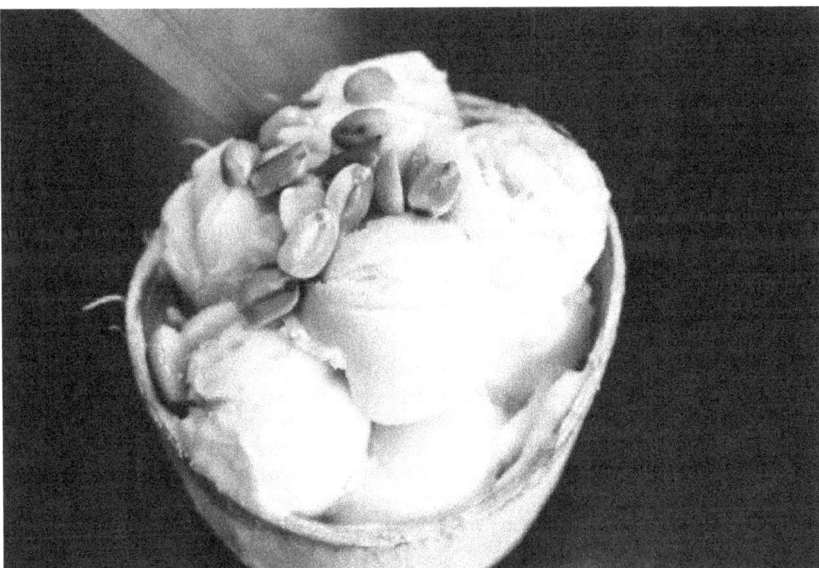

SERVES: 2
PREPARATION TIME: 15-20 min
COOLING TIME: 2-3 hours

INGREDIENTS:

Full fat coconut milk 1 can

Egg yolks 4

Vanilla extract (real) 4 tablespoons

Flavoring options:

Berries of your choice (chopped and blended) ½ cup

Coconut flakes ½ cup

Mint (finely chopped) ¼ cup

Orange, lemon or lime zest

Raw honey 3 tablespoons

Chocolate flakes or chips (dark chocolate) ¼ cup

METHOD:

1. Put some water in a large pot. Boil it and then reduce the heat to low.
2. Take a heat-proof bowl and place it over the pot so that a double boiler is formed.
3. Pour coconut milk in the bowl.
4. Put vanilla extract in the coconut milk.
5. Let the milk heat but do not let it boil. If you are using any other flavors, you can put them in this step only. If you want a chewy texture of dark chocolate, you can put the bits of it in later.
6. Put the eggs yolks in a bowl and whisk them.
7. Put a ladle of hot coconut milk into the egg mixture and whisk vigorously. Make sure that the eggs do not get cooked.
8. Gradually, add 2-3 ladles of hot milk into the egg mixture and keep whisking.
9. The egg mix has to be slowly poured into the double boiler in this step. Whisk the mixture again.
10. Keep whisking for a few minutes so that thick custard is formed.

11. Take care that the mixture does not get heated up too much and it does not come into contact with the water underneath.
12. Remove the custard from the heat once it is ready.
13. Once the custard is cool enough to handle, you can add more flavors if you want.

FREEZING:

1. Put the mixture in a bowl to cool in the refrigerator before freezing.
2. Put the mixture in a baking dish and place it in the freezer.
3. As mentioned above, you need to stir the custard every half an hour for 2-3 hours till it has frozen properly.
4. Serve with mint, berries, coconut flakes, coconut milk or any of your favorite flavors.

Filling Apple Fritters

Now you already know that you do not have to say goodbye to your favorite desserts because of your Paleo diet. You just have to experiment with a few things. Mix and match some ingredients here and there and yaayyy!! There you go with some mouth watering desserts.

In this recipe also, we have made a dessert out of apples. It is easy to make, delicious, as well as healthy. You can make it for any occasion. Think of incorporating them into your Christmas dinners. Think of some unique things that you can combine with these apple fritters. You never know, you might be the next chef writing a Paleo recipe book!

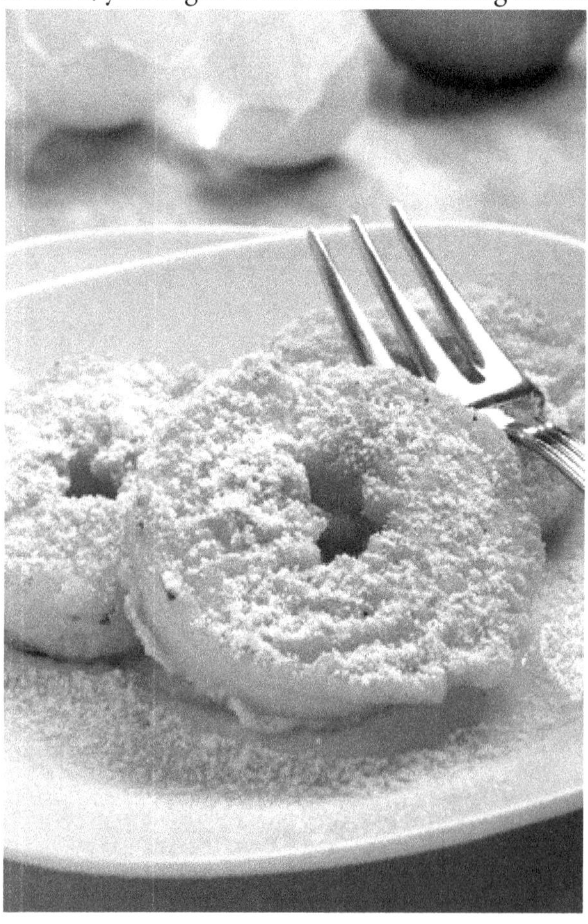

SERVES: 2
PREPARATION TIME: 15 min
INGREDIENTS:
Coconut flour ¼ cup
Arrowroot powder ¼ cup
Sea salt ¼ teaspoon
Whisked eggs 3 large
Maple syrup ¼ cup
Apple (cored, sliced and peeled) 1
Olive oil 3 cups (or less, for frying)
METHOD:

1. Take a medium sized bowl, and mix arrowroot powder, salt and coconut flour.
2. Mix maple syrup and eggs separately.
3. Combine the flour and eggs mixtures properly.
4. Cut ¼ inch apple rings. Dip into the batter.
5. Pour 2 inches of oil into a frying pan and heat.
6. Fry the battered apple rings for about 2 minutes on each side.
7. When the rings are fried well, take them out on a paper towel kept on a tray.
8. Serve with cinnamon sugar and ice-cream.

No-Bake Coconut Bars

Yes, it's true. You can make a dessert bar without baking. These coconut bars are absolutely addictive. Let's not forget to mention the fact that these can be prepared in just 10 minutes! And you do not have to be a robot to accomplish that!

Try these yummy coconut bars once and you would not be able to resist serving them to your guests again next time. Actually, they are best for those buddies who don't call before coming over, but just knock on the door at lunch time and say; "Hi!" You can prepare something for dessert in no time. While you have lunch, your dessert will be ready in your fridge.

SERVES: 2

PREPARATION TIME: 10 min

COOLING TIME: 2 hours

INGREDIENTS:

Unsweetened coconut (shredded) 1 cup

Agave nectar or maple syrup ¼ cup

Coconut oil (virgin) 1 tablespoon

Vanilla extract (pure) ½ teaspoon

Salt 1/8 teaspoon

Chocolate chips (optional) as much as you want

METHOD:

1. Put all the ingredients in a blender or food processor and pulse until they are combined well. You can keep a coarse texture.
2. Take out the mixture and press it in a small square container.
3. Chill in fridge.
4. When they have cooled properly, cut it into square pieces.
5. Serve with the chocolate chips topping.

See, we told you. It's ready in 10 minutes!

Paleo Bites of Brownie

Brownies are everyone's favorite. From kids to elders, everyone wants to grab the biggest portion of a brownie. And what more do you want when you have a healthy option for sweets? This brownie recipe is not just for Paleo lovers. Anybody can enjoy these sweet balls. Extremely easy and a real time-saver, these brownies with coconut coating are just so addictive.

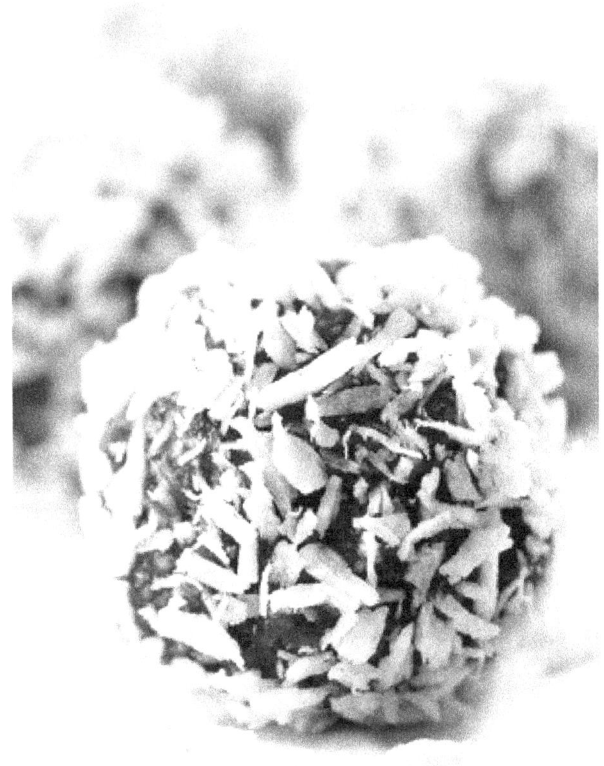

MAKES: 12 balls (1 inch)
PREPARATION TIME: 20 min
INGREDIENTS:

Walnut halves/pieces 2/3 cup
Cocoa powder (unsweetened) 1/3 cup
Pitted Mejdool dates 15-20
Vanilla extract 1 tablespoon
Coconut milk 2 tablespoons
Sweetener (agave, honey, maple syrup) (optional)
Unsweetened coconut (shredded) 2/3 cup
METHOD:

1. Put coconut in a food processor and pulse for about 30 seconds. Stop when you see that coconut has turned into crumbs.
2. Take the coconut crumbs out of the food processor and keep them covered.
3. Take a bowl of warm water and put pitted dates in it to soften for a minute or two.
4. Put cocoa powder (unsweetened) and walnuts in the food processor. Pulse to form coarse crumbs. Do not overdo the pulse otherwise you will end up making butter.
5. Drain the dates. Put them in the food processor along with walnut cocoa crumbs. Add vanilla extract.
6. Pulse the food processor to combine the ingredients.
7. If you find that the mixture does not combine well, it is because it needs a liquid to bind it. Coconut milk acts as a binder in such recipes.
8. Add half a tablespoon of coconut milk to the mixture and pulse. Keep adding half tablespoons of coconut milk until you find that the mixture has reached the correct consistency to make balls.
9. The right consistency is when the mixture sticks to the center of the food processor in the form of a big ball.
10. If you have added more milk than required and the mixture

has become runny, you can add a tablespoon or more of cocoa powder. It will come back to a dough.

11. Take out the dough into a bowl and cover it with plastic wrap.
12. Refrigerate the mixture for minimum of 2 hours. It is easier to work with cold dough.

MAKING BALLS:

1. Take the dough out of the refrigerator. Taking one tablespoon at a time, make balls of the dough using your hands. You can moisten your hands using water to prevent the dough sticking to your hands.
2. Put the coconut crumbs in a shallow bowl. Roll the cocoa balls in the crumbs and press gently so that the crumbs stick to the balls.
3. Serve chilled.

Truffles with Chocolate, Coconut and Coffee

By now, you must have got an idea that you do not have to wait for the non-Paleo products to savor the taste of delicious desserts. Here's another Paleo dessert that you can quickly make and enjoy with your loved ones. Make it, share it and enjoy it.

You can experiment with this recipe with as many flavors as you want. Since the base is coconut butter, it goes well with any kind of flavor.

An interesting experiment is to add a piece of fruit to each compartment of the tray before you pour the mixture in. The fruit bite adds a boost to the chocolate bite. Strawberry, mango or any fruit you can think of can be added to the tray. When it pops out and melts in your mouth, you are going to reach another world of heavenliness.

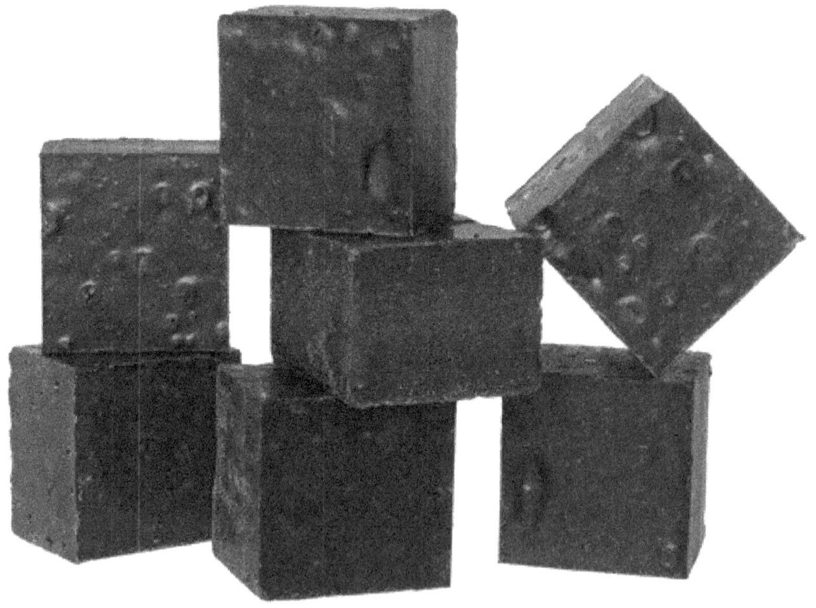

MAKES: 12 balls (1 inch)
PREPARATION TIME: 20 min
INGREDIENTS:
Coconut butter ½ cup

Dark cocoa powder 3 tablespoon
Ground coffee 1 tablespoon
Coconut flakes (unsweetened) 1 tablespoon
Raw honey ½ teaspoon
Coconut oil (virgin) 1 tablespoon

METHOD:

1. If you find that the coconut butter in the can is not soft, melt it in the microwave so that you can achieve a consistency that can be stirred with a fork.
2. Put all the ingredients in a bowl and mix using a fork.
3. Pick your favorite ice cube tray. Pour ¼ teaspoon of virgin coconut oil in the cups.
4. Spread the oil evenly. Basically, you have to grease the tray so that the chocolate chunks can pop out easily later.
5. Pour a spoonful of mixture into the cups (1 spoon for each cup).
6. Pat the mixture with a fork to flatten it.
7. Keep the tray in the freezer for a few hours. 4-5 hours are sufficient.
8. When you want to serve them, take them out 15-20 minutes beforehand.
9. Add any topping of your choice if you want.
10. Serve in a beautiful plate with a scoop of ice-cream.

<u>Conclusion</u>

How are you feeling now? After you have read some of the amazingly healthy and delicious recipes you can make while on the Paleo diet plan, you must be feeling positive about changing your diet. When I was writing this book, I just felt like rushing to the supermarket, grabbing the basic ingredients of Paleo recipes and making some of them. Being an expert at many of the Paleo recipes, I still feel new to this concept. There is so much to learn in this relatively new concept of lifestyle that you never get tired of cooking one thing or the other.

Paleo cooking does not require much expertise. Our old ancestors from the Stone Age weren't good cooks you see! Lol! If they could cook without any hi-tech cooking tools and instruments, why can't you? Forget the stigma attached to being an amateur to cooking. There is no such thing as a new cook. You can start cooking from anywhere you want. I would suggest beginning your Paleo journey with cooking desserts. Yes, start from the end of the book. It is the easiest part of this book. And when you think that you are at ease in the kitchen, you can try your hands at some of the other recipes too.

Now, for the expert cooks, I would say that you must have tried a lot of regular recipes. So it's a good time to bring a positive change in your eating habits and bring the wonderful Paleo cuisines to your platter. Since you already know how to cook, I would not suggest to you where to start from. Since you have read the book, you can pick up any recipe you want and just start cooking.

This is just a small book of Paleo cooking. There are a lot more recipes that I wanted to incorporate. But, I could not. I had to control myself. Anyway, you can still explore the world of Paleo. Keep experimenting with the recipes. You can add or subtract any ingredient you want. There are no hard and fast rules in cooking. While you are working in kitchen, you can accidentally discover many things that are never written in the books. Include them in your methods and share with others. That is the best way to learn while you teach. Happy cooking!

The Paleo Slow Cooker

The Ultimate Paleo Crock-Pot Cookbook for
Busy People
By: Emily Simmons

Table of Contents

<u>Slow cooker lasagna</u>
<u>Crockpot smashed sweet potato</u>
<u>Stuffed bell peppers</u>
<u>Gingerbread apple pudding cake</u>
<u>Choco-peanut nuggets</u>
<u>Conclusion</u>

Introduction

Some people think that *slow cooker* implies that you have to sit and wait for the food to get ready. But, there is no need to keep your head in your hands and wait for long hours when the aroma is spreading in your house and all you can do is wait! The best thing is to dump the ingredients in and forget about them for a few hours. You may even go to the office or the market or spend your day anywhere you want.

When you come home, a sumptuous and delicious meal will be waiting for you. The beauty of using the slow cooker is that you do not have to make much effort, but the outcomes are beyond expectations. But, if you do make some endeavor, there is no chance that your recipe will come out average. After all, cooking for hours must pay!

Paleo Diet Lovers: *The Ultimate Paleo Crock-Pot Cookbook for Busy People* deals with paleo friendly recipes which can be cooked in a crockpot. Most of these recipes consist of meat in various forms and a few desserts as well. This is so because the time taken by the slow cookers suits meat dishes best.

In the initial part of the book, you will find details about slow cooker methods and equipment and how the method works. You will also find suggestions as to which meat portions you should buy for slow cooking. Moreover, all the recipes mentioned in the book are tried and tested and you can modify them according to the slow cooker equipment you have in your kitchen.

Enjoy getting started on your new journey with slow cooking and you will get addicted to it.

Good luck!

Section 1

<u>**The Basics**</u>

Chapter 1

What is Slow Cooking?

You must be wondering what the point is of cooking food when you can do the same in just a few minutes and have equally delicious meals. The essence of slow cooking is that it gives you juicy, tender foods to savor every time. That is why it is worth spending some time with the preparation and the rest will be taken care of by the slow cooker.

Slow cooking is a method of cooking which gives you luscious meals with minimum effort. Moreover, this method is also budget-friendly. You need to buy sturdy cuts of different meats for this method so that they can bear the amount of heat over hours and you'll get flavorsome, hearty meals in the end. Although the cooking time is longer with this technique, the slow-cooked recipes call for relatively less time for preparation. After preparation, you can leave them to simmer on their own.

The advantage of the slow cooker method is that you'll save on the time of washing piles of pots and dishes because all the ingredients are cooked in one pot.

There are plenty of methods for cooking food slowly: simmer the food in a stockpot, bake the ingredients in a casserole inside the oven, or you can use specialized slow cooker devices like pressure cookers or electric slow cookers. We will explain all these methods later.

Chapter 2

Slow Cooking Methods and Equipment

Equipment for slow cooking

There is just one rule of thumb for slow cooking which you might know already- you need to combine vegetables, meat, seasonings and liquid in one pot only. However, the actual time taken by the recipes and their method of cooking varies widely depending upon the equipment you have. Have a look at this list of slow cooker equipment used widely all over the world:

Stockpot

This equipment consists of a large pot with a lid and two handles. It is typically made of aluminum or stainless steel. Stockpots come in various sizes. The larger ones often have more height than width.

The working of a stockpot: It is easy to work with stockpots. You can regard a stockpot as a large saucepan designed for holding larger quantities.

Why you should use a stockpot: When you cook food in this large pot over direct heat, you can adjust the amount of heat required. After the food is ready, you can take it out from the pot and let the cooking liquid remain inside to reduce over high heat. The sauce prepared in such a manner tastes delicious. You will find that stockpots are usually much larger than slow cooker appliances. Thus, you can cook a large quantity of food to freeze it in batches.

How you should buy it: You must buy a stockpot which has a heavy base so that it can bear the heat over several hours. It also helps to brown meat prior to putting in the other ingredients. The heavy base prevents the food from burning and sticking to the pot's base while it cooks.

Casserole

This is a low ovenproof dish with two handles and a tightly fitting lid. It may be made of ceramic, earthenware, glass, or any other material which is heat resistant.

The working of a casserole: For making a casserole, you need to brown the meat in a pan on a stovetop prior to placing it in the bowl with some liquid, herbs and vegetables. The bowl is then positioned in the oven with the lid on and the dish is slowly cooked until the meat becomes tender.

Why you should use a casserole: When you cook food in a casserole under indirect oven heat, you allow the heat to circulate around the bowl rather than focusing all the heat on the base. This reduces the chances of food getting burned at the base of the bowl and allows for more even cooking.

How you should buy a casserole: For slow cooking, you need to buy a casserole which is made of flameproof material like cast iron. You can use such a dish both inside the oven as well as on the stovetop. If the bowl is not flameproof, you can brown the meat in a frying pan on the stovetop first, and then the meat can be transferred to the dish for cooking in the oven.

Slow cooker/ crockpot

A slow cooker or a crockpot is an electrical device which contains a heatproof dish placed inside an outer casing made of metal. This dish can be removed whenever required. It also features a transparent lid along with temperature settings.

The working of a slow cooker: When food is cooked on the lowest setting of a slow cooker, it maintains an extremely low temperature such that it simmers very gently. This appliance takes more time in cooking than other methods of slow cooking. The device takes heat from the sides and thus the pot needs to be filled till half or three quarters. You can also use a slow cooker to keep the prepared food warm until you serve it.

Why you should use a slow cooker: This is a very convenient appliance to use. You can put all the ingredients in the pot and leave them to cook for several hours, even overnight. Since the heat is low, there are hardly any chances that the food will get overcooked, dry out or burn.

How you should buy a slow cooker: You must look for a crockpot which has a removable pot. This will help you to clean the pot easily. Also, the heating elements of the appliance should be on the sides, and not only in the bottom.

Pressure cooker

This looks similar to a stockpot except for its lid. The lid of a pressure cooker is designed so that it gets locked onto the pot and creates a firm seal.

The working of a pressure cooker: When you place a pressure cooker over a high flame, the liquid in the pot boils to create steam. The steam is locked inside the cooker, the pressure starts building up and this process increases the boiling point of the liquid. There is a regulator on top of the lid which lets the excess steam out gradually to prevent accidents. Before you open the lid, it is important that you let the pressure inside the cooker out. Otherwise there is a chance that the superheated liquid will come out at very high pressure, creating a dangerous situation. Also, you must put in the right quantity of food and liquid to cook the food properly.

Why you should use a pressure cooker: A pressure cooker gives your food the same flavor as that of slow cooking techniques, but it takes much less time.

How you should buy a pressure cooker: Look for a pressure cooker with a heavy base. The pressure cookers these days are safer and easier to use than the traditional models. Also, it is better to use stovetop models because the electric models are relatively less convenient. They take more time to cook because of their lower temperature settings and have only a few safety features.

Chapter 3

A Guide to Buying Meat Cuts for Slow Cooking

You must buy sturdy cuts of meat for slow cooking. These tend to be the cheaper cuts, so you will not only have good value for your money, but these cuts also have much more flavor than the more expensive cuts. The process of slow cooking is gentle and it gradually dissolves the tough connective tissue so that the meat becomes juicy and tender. Moreover, if you purchase meat which is still on the bone, it will add even more flavor to add to your gravy.

You can use this guide to buy the best portions of meat for the purpose of slow cooking:

<u>Beef</u>

Round steak

Chuck steak

Blade steak

Fresh silverside

Topside

Boneless shin beef (gravy)

Skirt steak

<u>Veal</u>

shin slices of Osso bucco

<u>Lamb</u>

Boneless forequarter

Boneless shoulder

Shanks

Best neck chops

Neck chops

<u>Chicken</u>

Any piece of chicken like drumsticks or thigh pieces are good, particularly those pieces on the bone.

<u>Pork</u>

Forequarter chops

Diced shoulder
Pork neck

Chapter 4

Tips for Slow Cooking

The main beauty of slow cooking is that it is a really simple process. You just need to prepare the ingredients, put them into the slow cooker and hit the Start button. However, there is a fine line between a *good* meal out of your slow cooker and a *great* one. Try to keep these tips in mind when you are dealing with a slow cooker or a crockpot:

1. **Use an appropriate size**

Slow cookers come in a wide range of sizes ranging from as small as 1 quart to as big as 8.5 quarts. You must use the size of slow cooker mentioned in the recipe. If you do not have the exact size mentioned, you can proportionately increase or decrease the quantity of ingredients to suit the size of the cooker. This makes sure that the cooker is not left vacant or gets overfilled, and that the food gets cooked properly.

1. **Do not overfill**

If you do not overfill your slow cooker, it will be able to cook the food in the time mentioned in the recipe. Not overfilling also prevents the potential safety hazards. Most cookers are recommended to be filled up to two thirds of their total volume.

1. **Do not take the lid off**

Resist your temptation to take the lid off to have a "look" at the food. If you open the lid, the heat escapes and the process of cooking is further slowed down. Open it only 30-45 minutes prior to the low end of the cooking time to check for doneness.

1. **Plan the meals**

Working with slow cookers is definitely easy, but it does require some planning.

The night prior to cooking: Chop the vegetables, trim and cut the meat, measure the ingredients, prepare the sauce and refrigerate the ingredients in separate containers. Do not make the mistake of refrigerating the ingredients in the pot of a slow cooker. Otherwise the pot will take a long time to heat up and will further affect the cooking time of the food as well as its safety.

The morning of cooking: As per the recipe, put the ingredients into the cooker and reheat the sauce prior to adding it to the cooker. If you will not be at home when the food is ready, turn the Warm Setting of the cooker on.

1. Maximize flavor

If you have some spare time before dumping the ingredients into the slow cooker, you can brown the vegetables and meat in a skillet prior to adding them to the slow cooker. Then, you can also deglaze the skillet and put the caramelized bits into the slow cooker. This will give your meal a rich texture and flavor which cannot be attained only by slow cooking.

1. Look for the temperature

It is definitely convenient to work with a slow cooker, but you must keep in mind the safety hazards of the slow cooker. The range of temperature between 40°-140° F comes into the danger zone because bacteria thrive in this range. Do not keep the food in this range for an excessively long time. To avoid bacteria multiplying, do not add frozen food into the cooker. You can only refrigerate the ingredients you have arranged in different containers, not freeze them. Also, before you add the liquids to the cooker, simmer them to quick-start the cooking process.

Do not ever try to cook a complete piece of roast or chicken in the slow cooker. They do not cook thoroughly this way. Cut the meat into smaller pieces which can then be easily cooked in the slow cooker.

Section 2
Slow Cooker Recipes
Chicken Musakhan

Indulge in this Middle Eastern chicken dish without any guilt. It looks heavenly and tastes delicious as well. The addition of sumac powder to the chicken makes it extraordinary.

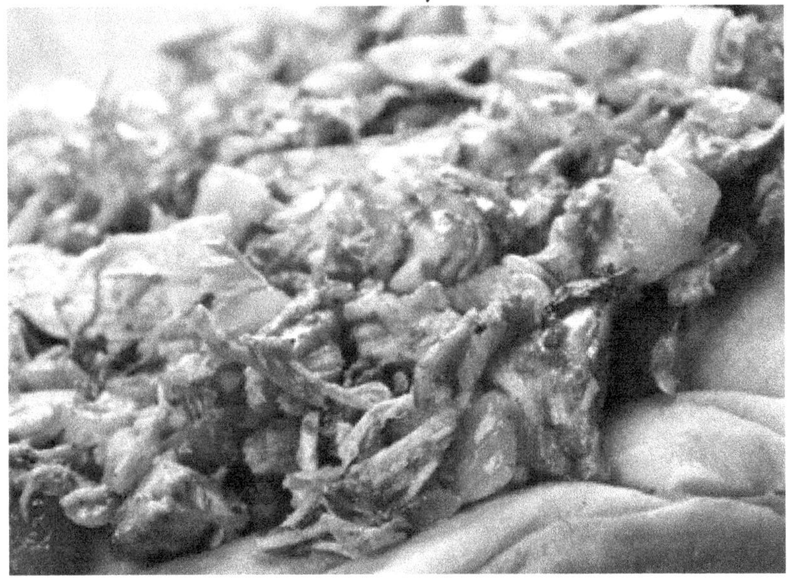

SERVES: 6
PREPARATION TIME: 15 minutes
COOKING TIME: 6 hours
INGREDIENTS:

Skinless boneless chicken thighs 2.5 pounds

Thinly sliced onions 2

Olive oil 1.5 tablespoon

Sumac powder (ground) 0.5 ounce **or**

Paprika powder (1 teaspoon) with lemon juice (half teaspoon)

Cinnamon 1 teaspoon

All spice mix (ground) ¼ teaspoon

Ground cloves ¼ teaspoon

Saffron 1 big pinch
Pine nuts a handful
Fresh mint, chopped 2 tablespoons
Salt as per taste
Pepper as per taste

METHOD:

1. Take a large bowl which is microwave safe and put in the onions, sumac powder, olive oil, cinnamon, cloves powder, all spice mix, and saffron. Mix the ingredients and microwave them for 2.5 minutes. Take out the bowl and stir. Microwave it again for another 2.5 minutes.

Alternatively, you can also sauté the ingredients in a pan. Put the onions and oil in a pan and sauté. Add the spices and stir till the onions are brown. The microwave method is a shortcut.

1. Thaw the chicken and dump it into the crock pot. Season it liberally with pepper and salt. Put in the mixture of onions and stir. The chicken should be snuggled in the onions mixture.
2. Turn on the slow cooker and cook for 6 hours on low. Before serving, sauté some pine nuts in a little olive oil until browned over medium low heat. Chop the mint finely.
3. You can add more pepper and salt if you would like to. Take out the chicken and put it into a serving dish. Top it with pine nuts and mint.

<u>Pork Ribs</u>

The seasonings on these pork ribs work amazingly well and gives them a special aroma. If you are a pork fan, this dish will be a real treat for you.

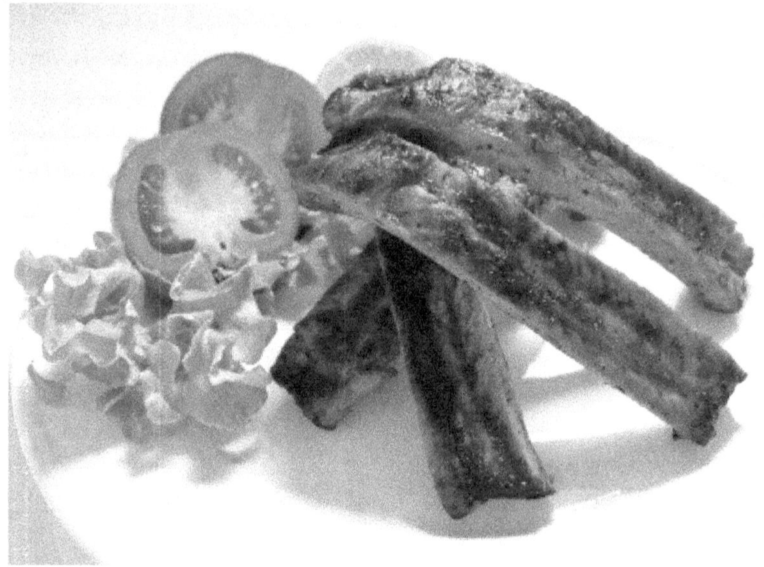

SERVES: 6
PREPARATION TIME: 1-night soaking + 15 minutes
COOKING TIME: 6 hours
INGREDIENTS:
Pork ribs (pasture raised) 3-4 pounds
White vinegar 2-4 cups
Pure water 1-2 cups
Sea salt 1-2 cups
Sea salt 1 teaspoon
Apple cider or rice wine vinegar 2 tablespoons
Tamari (wheat free) or coconut aminos 3 tablespoons
Extra sea salt as per taste
Freshly ground black pepper as per taste
Garlic powder ½ - 1 teaspoon

Five spice powder 1 teaspoon

Sliced raw tomato 1

METHOD:

1. Mix water and vinegar in the ratio of 1:2. Cover the pork ribs with this mixture and mix with one teaspoon sea salt. Soak it in a bowl overnight.
2. Drain the ribs next morning.
3. Sprinkle the ribs with generous amounts of black pepper, garlic powder and salt on both sides.
4. Give a heavy coating of 5 spice powder on both sides of the ribs. The meat should be thoroughly coated with the orange colored powder.
5. Rub these seasonings gently into both sides of the ribs.
6. Position the ribs standing on the ends in the pot of slow cooker. Let them lean a little.
7. Add tamari or coconut aminos and rice wine vinegar to the base of slow cooker.
8. Set the slow cooker on high and cook the ribs for 4-6 hours. Since there is not much liquid in the slow cooker, the ribs are getting roasted, not stewed. Thus, you must keep your attention on them so that they do not get too dry.
9. Serve with a few slices of raw tomatoes.

<u>Slow Cooker Roast</u>

Beef prepared with this recipe is deliciously aromatic. The goodness of vegetables and semi-cooked cauliflower gives a unique taste to the beef. Just take it out of the crockpot and serve.

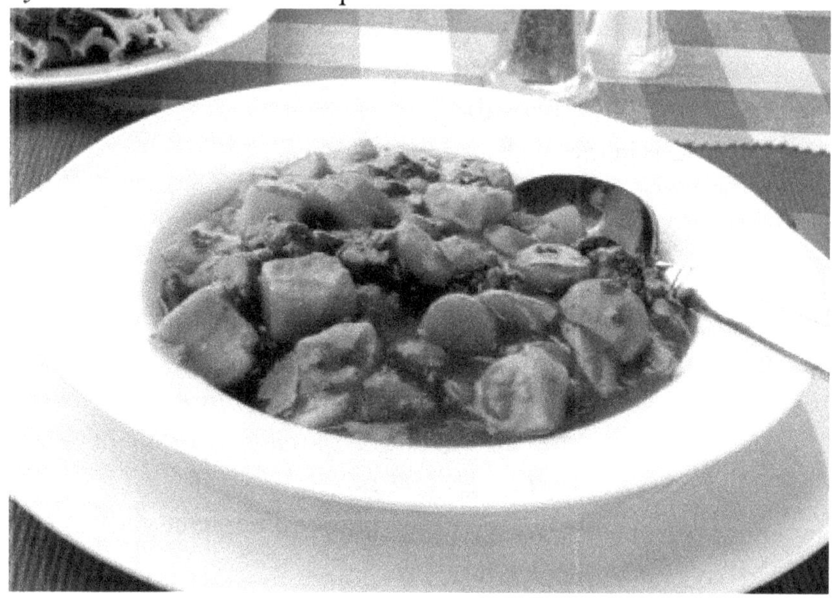

SERVES: 6

PREPARATION TIME: 15 minutes

COOKING TIME: 8 hours 20 minutes

INGREDIENTS:

Beef chuck roast 4 pounds

Olive oil or coconut oil 1 tablespoon

Good quality red wine 1 cup

Garlic cloves 4

Fresh thyme 10 sprigs

Bay leaf 1

Peeled and chunked carrots 1 large or 2 small

Chunked celery ribs 2

Chunked onions 1 small
Cauliflower (cut in florets) 1 small head
Salt as per taste
Pepper (freshly ground) as per taste
METHOD:

1. Switch on the slow cooker and set it to low. Season the beef with a liberal amount of pepper and salt.
2. Preheat a skillet or a large sauté pan over medium high temperature. Add olive oil to the skillet and swirl to coat it.
3. Add beef to the skillet and sear it. In a while, a brown crust will be formed on the beef. Flip the beef to the other side and sear it too. keep flipping the beef so that it is seared on all sides.
4. Remove the beef from the skillet and put it into the slow cooker.
5. While the skillet is still hot, pour red wine into it to deglaze it. The wine will come to the boil quickly, while loosening some of the morsels from the skillet. Use a wooden spatula to scrape out as much as possible. Pour this blend of red wine over the beef.
6. Add thyme, bay leaves and garlic to the slow cooker. These ingredients must cover every part of the beef.
7. Put the remaining vegetables to the slow cooker, keeping aside the florets of cauliflower. Season the beef with some pepper and salt. Push these ingredients on the sides of the beef. As the vegetables are on the side, the beef tastes better as it cooks. The vegetables and beef will shrink as they cook and their juices with give the meat an amazing flavor.
8. Cover the slow cooker with its lid and let the ingredients simmer gently for 8 hours.
9. After the time is over, put cauliflower florets into the cooker

and push them under the liquid. Season using some pepper and salt and cover again with the lid. Cook for another 20 minutes.

10. Take out into a bowl and serve.

<u>Pad Thai Chicken with Vegetable Noodles</u>

Completely healthy noodles made of zucchini, and chicken garnished with green onions and cashews is an absolute delight. This Pad Thai chicken cooks in a relatively shorter time in a small crockpot.

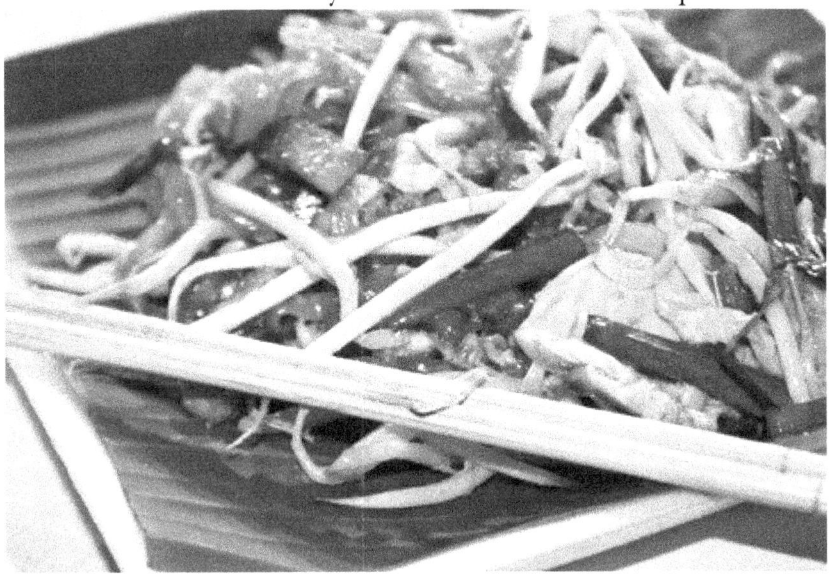

SERVES: 6
PREPARATION TIME: 15-20 minutes
COOKING TIME: 3-4 hours
INGREDIENTS:

Chicken breasts or thighs 2-3 pounds

Zucchini 2 medium

Carrot 1 large

Bean sprouts 2/3 cup

Green onions 1 small bunch (for garnish and sauce)

Coconut milk 1 cup

Chicken stock 1 cup

Sunbutter (sunflower seed butter) 2 tablespoons, heaped

Coconut aminos 1 tablespoon

Fish sauce 2 teaspoons

Powdered ginger 2 teaspoons
Garlic, minced and smashed 2 cloves
Cayenne pepper 1 teaspoon
Red pepper flakes 1 teaspoon
Salt as per taste
Pepper as per taste
Chopped cashews (optional) for garnish
Chopped cilantro (optional) for garnish
METHOD:

1. Season the chicken with pepper and salt and some ginger powder and cayenne pepper.
2. Brown the chicken in a skillet made of cast iron to get maximum flavor. You can skip this step if you do not have time.
3. Add chicken stock and coconut milk to the pot of a 4 quart slow cooker set on low. Stir well. If you are using full fat coconut milk, ensure that you combine the chicken stock with coconut milk.
4. Add coconut aminos, sunbutter, garlic, ginger, fish sauce, 2 green onions (chopped) including their whites, red pepper and cayenne.
5. Mix well so that the sunbutter gets completely dissolved.
6. Put the chicken into the liquid mixture in the pot.
7. Using a spiral slicer, make noodles out of the zucchinis. Wash the bean sprouts and shred the carrots.
8. Take a bowl and put in the zucchini noodles, bean sprouts and shredded carrots and combine them well.
9. Nestle the vegetables on top of the chicken and liquid in the crockpot. Press them slightly so that the vegetables come out steamed. We do not want to stew them.
10. Cook the ingredients for 3-4 hours. If you are using a bigger

slow cooker, say 6-quart, do not cook for over 6 hours.

11. Before serving, remove the noodles and keep them aside, straining them of any liquid.

12. Remove the chicken and debone it, chopping the chicken into strips. Pour some liquid from the slow cooker onto the chicken and combine well.

13. Place the chicken with sauce on the noodles in a plate and garnish with chopped cilantro, chopped cashews and green onions.

<u>Shredded Beef with Green Chile Cabbage Bowl</u>

The colorful red cabbage gives a beautiful color to this recipe for beef. While the beef gets prepared in the slow cooker, half an hour before serving you can prepare the dressing and there you are! Ready with a mouthwatering lunch!

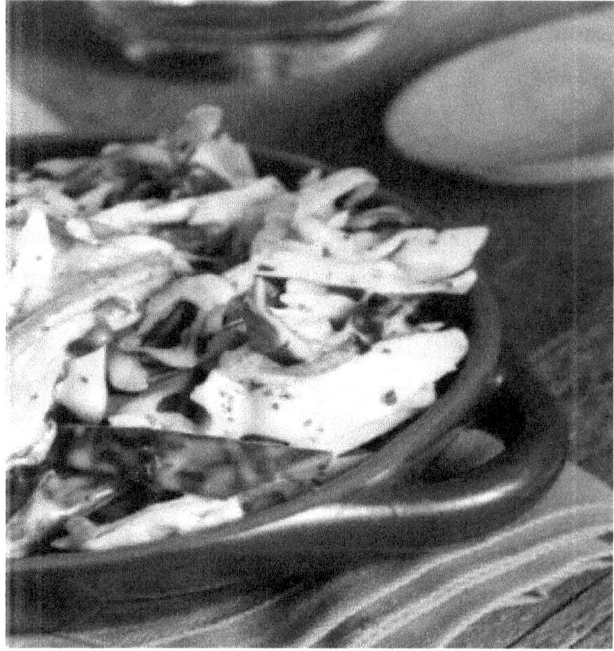

SERVES: 6
PREPARATION TIME: 30 minutes
COOKING TIME: 3-4 hours
INGREDIENTS (for beef):
Beef chuck roast, stripped 2 pounds
Taco seasoning 1 tablespoon
Olive oil 2-3 teaspoon
Green chilies, diced, with juice 2 cans
INGREDIENTS (for dressing and cabbage slaw):
Green cabbage 1 small head
Red cabbage ½ small head
Green onions, thinly sliced ½ cup
Light mayonnaise 6 tablespoons
Lime juice 4 teaspoons
Green Tabasco sauce 2 teaspoons
INGREDIENTS (for Avocado Salsa):
Diced avocados 2 large
Poblano pepper 1 medium
Lime juice, freshly squeezed 1 tablespoon
Olive oil, extra virgin 1 tablespoon
Cilantro, finely chopped ½ cup **or**
Green onion, finely sliced ¼ cup (if you do not like cilantro)
METHOD:

1. Use a 3.5-quart crock pot or a little smaller than that.
2. Remove all the visible undesirable parts or fat from the chuck roast. Cut the beef into thick strips. You can use the scraps later to make beef stock.
3. Rub the beef strips with taco seasoning.
4. Take a large and heavy frying pan and heat some oil. Brown the beef in it on all sides. As you already know, browning adds significant flavor to the meat.

5. Put the browned beef in the crockpot and add the canned juice and green chilies. Cook these ingredients for 3-4 hours on high. The beef should come apart easily. If you prefer, you can cook it on low for 6-8 hours.
6. Take out the beef and place on a cutting board, straining the liquid. Shred the meat apart using two forks. Put the beef back into the crockpot so that it may absorb the liquid.
7. Shred the cabbage finely. Cut the green onions into slices.
8. Whisk the lime juice, green Tabasco sauce and mayonnaise together for a dressing. Adjust the ingredients if you want to make it creamier or more tangy.
9. Combine the green onions and cabbage with the dressing.
10. Peel the avocado and dice it. Put it into a bowl and pour lime juice over. Toss them to combine. Put finely sliced green onions or chopped cilantro, and the Poblano pepper into this bowl. Drizzle in some olive oil and toss again.
11. Now, to assemble a serving bowl per person, place a layer of the salad in the bottom. Place a liberal quantity of beef from the slow cooker on top. Then top everything with two tablespoons of avocado salsa.

1.

Chicken Mole Crock Pot

The tangy taste of jalapenos and avocado on top of chicken lets you enjoy the meat even more. A perfect meal with a glass of wine after a long day.

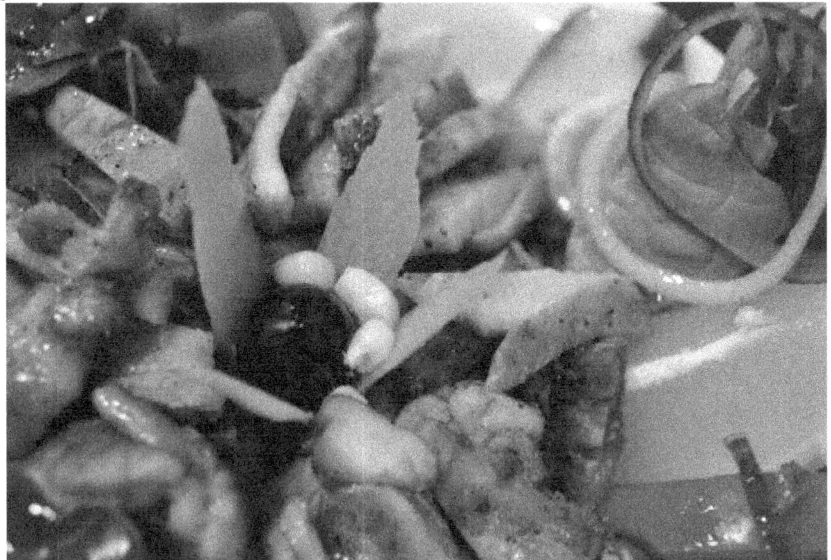

SERVES: 6
PREPARATION TIME: 30 minutes
COOKING TIME: 3-4 hours
INGREDIENTS:

Chicken breasts 2 pounds

Salt as per taste

Pepper as per taste

Ghee 2 tablespoon

Chopped onion 1 medium

Minced and crushed garlic 4 cloves

Peeled, seeded, chopped whole tomatoes 6-7

Mexican chili peppers, chopped and rehydrated 5

Almond butter ¼ cup

Sea salt 1 teaspoon
Dark chocolate 2.5 ounces
Cumin powder 1 teaspoon
Cinnamon powder ½ teaspoon
Chili powder ½ teaspoon
Cilantro, chopped for garnish
Avocado, chopped for garnish
Jalapeno, chopped for garnish

METHOD:

1. Sprinkle pepper and salt generously on chicken.
2. Take a sauté pan on high heat and put ghee in.
3. After the ghee has melted, put chicken in the pan and brown it from all sides. You can do this step in batches.
4. After browning all the chicken pieces, put them into the slow cooker.
5. In the same sauté pan, add onions and sauté them till they become translucent.
6. Add garlic. Combine it with onions and sauté for 2 minutes.
7. Put this mixture into the slow cooker.
8. Put chili peppers, tomatoes, dark chocolate, almond butter, spices and salt into the cooker.
9. Set the cooker on low and cook for 4-6 hours. The chicken should become tender and come apart easily.
10. Take the chicken out onto a plate and garnish with cilantro, jalapeno and avocado. Serve hot.

Salmon Head Delicious Soup

The beauty of this wonderfully rich soup is that you have a lot of things to enjoy while slurping it. You can chew the pieces of salmon meat along with the vegetables and zucchini noodles. Your stomach may feel full after just one bowl, but your heart will definitely crave for more!

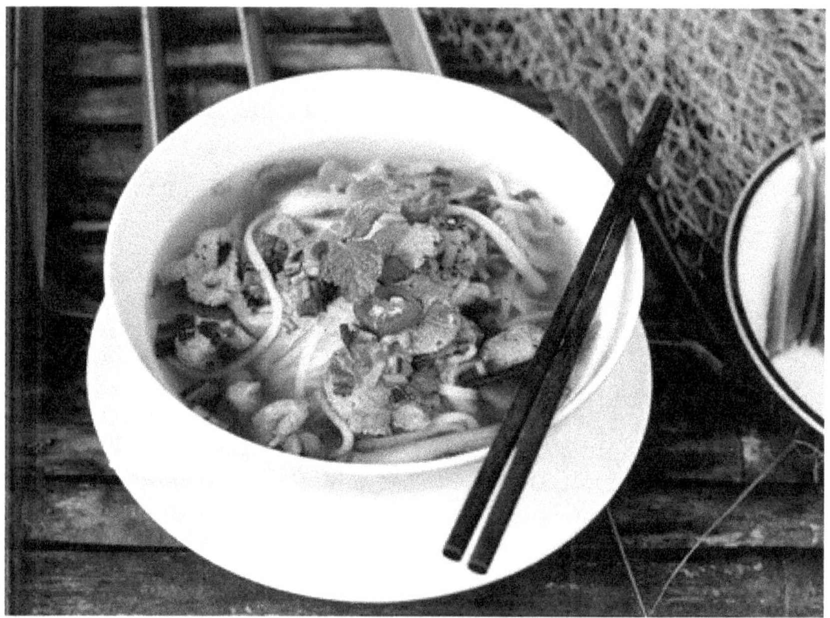

SERVES: 4-6
PREPARATION TIME: 30 minutes
COOKING TIME: 3 hours
INGREDIENTS:
Salmon head 1
Salmon tail 1
Some more pieces of salmon
Sliced onion 1 small
Minced garlic 1 bulb
Wakame (edible seaweed) 1 cup
3-inch piece slivered ginger 1 piece and

Peeled, minced ginger 1 tablespoon
Mirin ¼ cup or (¼ cup coconut vinegar)
Coconut aminos or tamari ¼ cup
Spiraled zucchini noodles 3 zucchinis
Chilies and chives for garnish

METHOD:

1. Put salmon tails and heads and the extra pieces of the fish along with the slivered ginger in the slow cooker. Cover them with water. You don't have to peel the ginger if you wish for this step.
2. Set the slow cooker on high and cook for 1.5 to 2 hours.
3. Sieve the broth and pull the meat.
4. Put back the broth and deboned, shredded meat into the slow cooker. Add onions, garlic, minced ginger, mirin, tamari and wakame.
5. Heat the soup a little but do not let it come to boil. Let it cook for 20 minutes.
6. During this time, you can spiral the zucchini noodles.
7. Add these noodles to the slow cooker and let them cook for another 10 to 15 minutes.
8. When the zucchinis become tender, serve the soup into serving bowls. Garnish with chilies and chives.

Butternut Soup

The butternut squash soup comes out a beautiful rich color and adds a loveliness to your meals. If you want to have a light meal, you can have only this soup and stay full for some time.

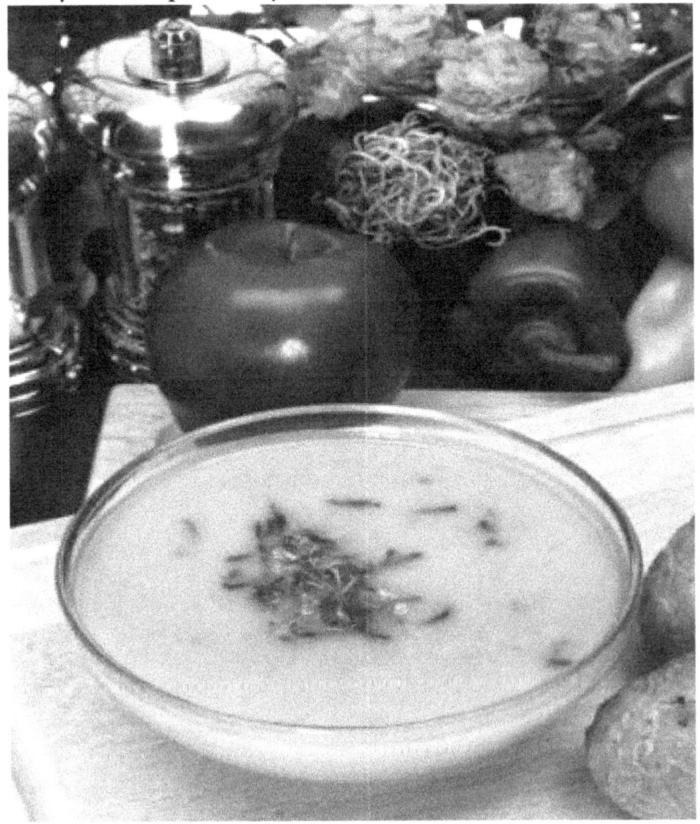

SERVES: 6
PREPARATION TIME: 15 minutes
COOKING TIME: 8 hours
INGREDIENTS:
Raw walnuts ½ cup
Raw almonds ½ cup
Peeled, cubed butternut squash 1 medium
Peeled, cubed apples 2

Cinnamon 1 teaspoon
Nutmeg ½ teaspoon
Coconut sugar 1 tablespoon (adjust if you want more)
Coconut milk 1 cup
TOPPINGS:
Desiccated coconut
Coconut milk
Maple syrup

METHOD:

1. Soak the walnuts and almonds in filtered water. Add a pinch of sea salt. Let them soak for at least 12 hours. You need to plan in advance for this step.
2. Rinse the nuts using filtered water.
3. Put the nuts in a small jar of food processor and blend. The nuts should be blended until the consistency of flour is attained.
4. Put the apples, butternut squash, cinnamon, nutmeg, coconut sugar, coconut milk and ground nuts in a 6-quart slow cooker.
5. Set the cooker on low and cook for 8 hours.
6. When the butternut is ready, mash it using a potato masher into the consistency you prefer.
7. Top it with some toppings and serve it in your favorite bowl.

Wraps with Pulled Chicken

You need to wait a bit for these delicious crunchy wraps of lettuce and chicken. The fresh crunchiness of the lettuce leaves contrasts well with the softness of the chicken.

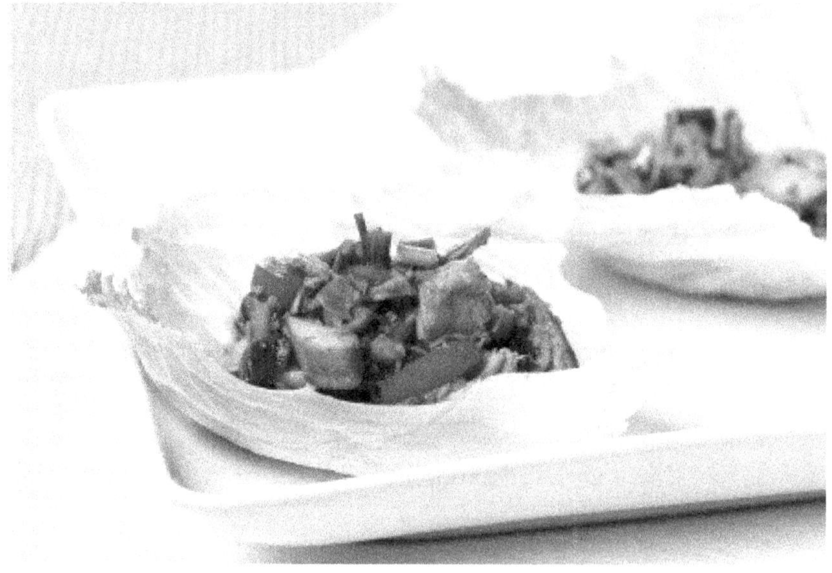

SERVES: 2
PREPARATION TIME: 10 minutes
COOKING TIME: 6 hours
INGREDIENTS:
Chicken breasts 2
Tomatoes 2
Red Onions 2
Garlic cloves 2
Honey 1 tablespoon
Basil 1 teaspoon
Chili powder 1 teaspoon
Whole cloves 1 teaspoon
Water 3 tablespoon
Lettuce leaves

Toothpicks
Salad of grated vegetables such as red cabbage and carrots
METHOD:

1. Cut the tomatoes and onions into small chunks.
2. Chop the garlic cloves finely.
3. Put the chicken breasts in the crockpot.
4. Add tomatoes, onions, garlic, honey, chili, basil, water and whole cloves over the chicken breasts.
5. Cook on low for at least 6 hours.
6. Remove the chicken breasts and pull the meat apart using two forks.
7. Put the meat back into the pot and stir all the ingredients together until they are well combined.
8. Spread spoonfuls of the mixture onto each lettuce leaf and sprinkle some lemon juice on top. Wrap the lettuce leaf over the filling and secure it in place using a toothpick.
9. Place the wrap on a plate along with the grated salad on the side.

Short Ribs with Ginger and Star Anise

Do you stay busy throughout the day but wait for a hearty meal of short ribs? Do not worry. This meal requires minimal preparation time and you are ready to go for a quick and fulfilling meal later on.

SERVES: 1

PREPARATION TIME: 10 minutes

COOKING TIME: 6 hours

INGREDIENTS:

Short rib beef 1

Red onions 2 small

Minced garlic cloves 2

Ground ginger 1 teaspoon

Star anise 2

Honey 1 tablespoon

Salt as per taste

Pepper as per taste

METHOD:

1. Crush the cloves of garlic and chop red onions.
2. Put beef rib into the pot of slow cooker.
3. Put garlic, onions, star anise, honey and ginger on top.
4. Pour in approximately 1 inch of water.
5. Set the slow cooker on auto, cover it with lid and let the ingredients cook for 6-8 hours.
6. When the beef rib is ready, season it with salt and pepper.
7. Serve with a salad of carrots, cucumber and cabbage.

<u>Crock Pot Beef with Kale and Root Veggies</u>

Freshly steamed kale leaves along with cut pieces of protein rich beef provide you with a sumptuous meal. This easy to cook recipe has all the qualities of a flavorsome, filling dinner.

SERVES: 2

PREPARATION TIME: 15 minutes

COOKING TIME: 6 hours

INGREDIENTS:

Chunks of braising beef steak 14 ounces

Chopped chunks of red onions 2

Chopped carrots 2 large

Swede, cut into chunks 2

Celeriac ½ (remove the skin and chop it into cubes)

Garlic cloves 6

Sea salt as per taste

Pepper as per taste

Water

Kale 2-3 cups

Potato any kind

METHOD:

1. Put beef steak into the slow cooker.
2. Put carrots, onions, celeriac, garlic and swede over the beef.
3. Season with pepper and salt.
4. Pour water in to a depth of about 2 inches. Do not fill the cooker pot completely.
5. Cook for about 6 hours on auto.
6. When the beef is ready to eat, place fresh kale leaves on top of it and put the lid back on. Let the kale steam for 5-10 minutes.
7. Serve in small bowls.

Slow Cooker Chili Chicken

This Mexican chili chicken is superbly easy and ridiculously delicious. You can have it with lettuce leaves or cauliflower rice. But, do not forget to get a superior salsa.

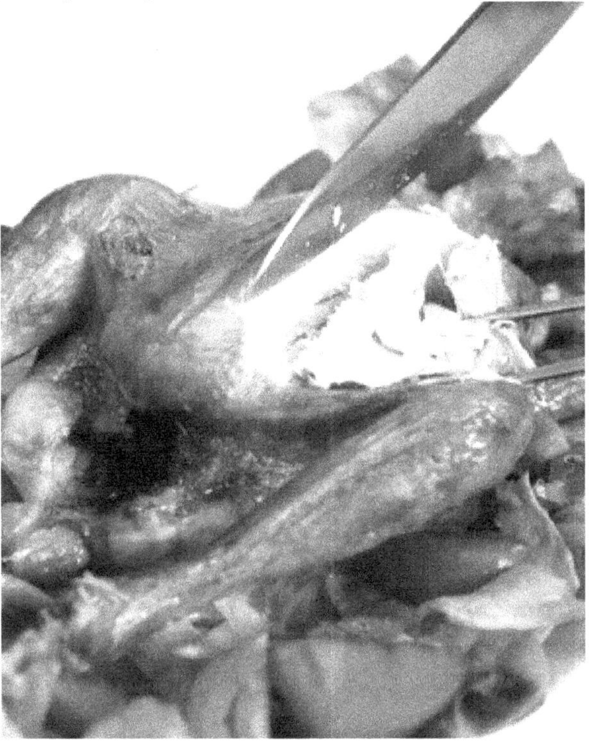

SERVES: 2
PREPARATION TIME: 15 minutes
COOKING TIME: 6 hours
INGREDIENTS:
Chicken thighs, boneless 6-8
16 ounces salsa 1 jar
16 ounces diced tomatoes 1 jar
Chopped yellow onion 1 medium
Chopped red pepper 1 large
Chili powder 2 tablespoons
Cauliflower rice or lettuce leaves for serving
Shredded cheese for topping
METHOD:

1. Dice chicken thigh meat and put it into the crockpot.
2. Sprinkle chili powder over the chicken and stir to ensure that the chicken is coated well with it.
3. Add all the vegetables. Stir well.
4. Pour salsa along with tomatoes over the mixture. Stir again.
5. Put the lid onto the cooker and set it on high. Cook for 4-6 hours and then cook again on 6-8 hours on the low setting. The longer it cooks, the better it will taste.
6. Serve the chicken over cauliflower rice on a plate. You can also serve it with lettuce leaves with a spoonful of guacamole. Top it with shredded cheese.

Crockpot Chili Pulled Pork

The freshness of green onions and avocados in this recipe contrast so well with the pork. Invest in the time taken by this pork and you will want to do it again and again.

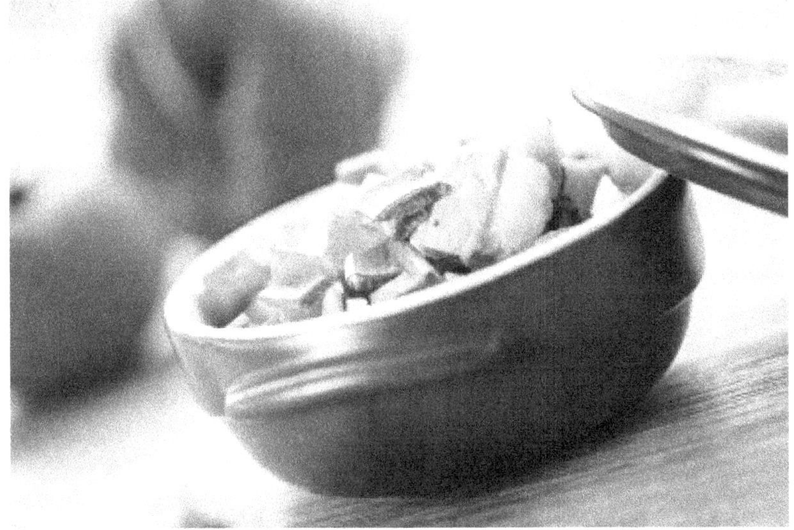

SERVES: 6-8
PREPARATION TIME: 10 minutes
COOKING TIME: 10 hours
INGREDIENTS:
Pork roast 2 pounds (trim excess fat)
Peeled garlic cloves 3
Hot sauce ½ cup
Smoked paprika 3 tablespoons
Garlic powder 2 tablespoons
Chili powder 2 tablespoons
Cumin 1 tablespoon
Cayenne pepper 2 teaspoons
Red pepper flakes 1 tablespoon (heaping)
Salt generous amount as you like
Diced yellow onions 2

Diced red bell pepper 1

Diced yellow bell pepper 1

2 cans of 14 ounces roasted tomatoes (fire roasted)

1 can of 14 ounce tomato sauce

Sliced avocado for garnish

Diced green onions for garnish

METHOD:

1. Put the pork roast in the slow cooker.

2. Make 3 holes in the pork with the point of a sharp knife and push the garlic cloves into them.

3. Pour some hot sauce over the pork.

4. Sprinkle garlic powder, paprika, chili powder, cumin seeds, red pepper flakes, salt and cayenne pepper over the roast.

5. Put diced peppers, onions, tomato sauce and tomatoes over the ingredients.

6. Cover the cooker with the lid and set it on low.

7. Cook for 8-10 hours.

8. Remove the pork and shred it, using to forks.

9. Remove to a serving dish and garnish with green onions and sliced avocado.

Roasted Cabbage and Beef Brisket

The roasted cabbage tastes amazingly delicious with beef brisket. Once you try this delicious dish you'll want to make it again and again.

SERVES: 6-8

PREPARATION TIME: 10 minutes

COOKING TIME: 10 hours

INGREDIENTS (Beef brisket):

Beef brisket, corned 2.5 pounds

Onion ½ medium

Carrot 1

Celery stalk 1

Beef or chicken stock 1 cup

INGREDIENTS (roasted cabbage or Brussel sprouts):

Green cabbage 1 head

Avocado oil 1 tablespoon

Salt as per taste

Pepper as per taste

METHOD (beef brisket):

1. Prepare the ingredients. Chop carrot, celery stalk and onion. Put them on the base of the slow cooker.

2. Pour beef or chicken stock over the vegetables.

3. Place beef brisket over the vegetables in the slow cooker.

4. Secure the slow cooker with a lid and set it on low. Cook for 6 to 8 hours.

METHOD (Roasted Cabbage or Brussel sprouts):

1. Preheat your oven to 450°F.

2. Cut the cabbage head into 8 wedges. Place them on a baking sheet (rimmed). You can also use Brussel sprouts and cut them into half.

3. Brush the cabbage wedges on both sides with avocado oil. Sprinkle pepper and salt over them to your taste.

4. Place the dish into the oven and roast for 25 to 30 minutes. Flip them after 15-20 minutes so that you get brown crispy edges.

5. Once done, remove the beef brisket from the crock pot onto a serving plate; place some of the vegetables on one side. Pour the juices from the crockpot over. Place the roasted cabbage on the other side of the plate and serve hot.

Coconut and Lemongrass Chicken Drumsticks

The marinade on the chicken drumsticks works wonders and has a unique taste of ginger and garlic. It is even better if you marinade the chicken for an hour or so before putting it into the slow cooker.

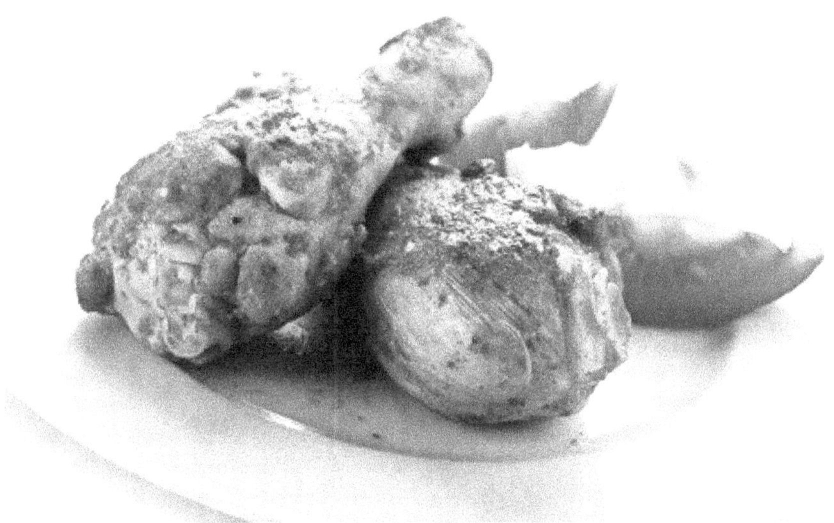

SERVES: 4-6
PREPARATION TIME: 20 minutes
COOKING TIME: 5 hours
INGREDIENTS:

Skinless chicken drumsticks 10

Fresh lemongrass 1 heavy stalk

Garlic cloves 4

Ginger, finely grated 2-inch piece

Coconut milk 1 cup

Red boat fish sauce 2 tablespoons

Coconut aminos 3 tablespoons

Five spice powder 1 teaspoon

Thinly sliced onion 1 large

Chopped, fresh scallions ¼ cup

  EMILY SIMMONS

Tomato wedges 2 tomatoes
Kosher salt as per taste
Ground pepper, freshly ground as per taste

METHOD:

1. Pull the skin off the drumsticks using a paper towel. You will find it easier to hold the slippery drumsticks after the skin is removed.
2. Put the chicken drumsticks in a bowl. Season them using pepper and salt.
3. Remove the rough bottoms and papery outer membrane of the lemongrass. Trim them to the lower 5 inches.
4. Put the garlic, ginger, fish sauce, coconut milk, five spice powder and coconut aminos into the blender jar. Pulse until the ingredients are made into a smooth sauce.
5. Pour the blended marinade onto the drumsticks in the bowl. Mix well so that the chicken is completely coated in the paste.
6. Once you're ready to cook, put the chopped onion into the slow cooker. Put the coated drumsticks in along with the marinade over the onions. Cook on low for 4-5 hours. Do not cook on high and beyond 5 hours. Check the seasonings and adjust if you want to.
7. Remove the drumsticks and put on a serving plate. Sprinkle chopped scallions on top, place tomato wedges on the side and serve.

<u>Slow Cooker Pork Tenderloin with Apple</u>
You'll still remember this delicious meal days after you've eaten it.
SERVES: 4-6
PREPARATION TIME: 20 minutes
COOKING TIME: 5 hours
INGREDIENTS:
Gala apples 4 organic
Pork tenderloin 2 pounds
Nutmeg powder as per taste
Raw honey 2 tablespoons
METHOD:

1. Core the apples and slice them into thin wedges.
2. Spread a layer of half of the apples on the base of the slow cooker, reserving the rest. Sprinkle some nutmeg powder over the apples.
3. Using a sharp knife, make deep slits in the pork at regular intervals.
4. Place one apple wedge in each of the slits of the tenderloins.
5. Place the pork tenderloins along with the apples over the apple layer already placed in the slow cooker.
6. Put any remaining slices of apples on top of the pork.
7. Sprinkle some nutmeg powder over the top.
8. Drizzle some fresh honey over if you want some extra sweetness.
9. Set the slow cooker on low, and cook for 8 hours.
10. Serve pork tenderloins right from the slow cooker to the plate.

Cashew Chicken

Top this slow cooked cashew chicken with beans or green onions, and serve it with all the juices from the crockpot. Your family will love this amazing meal.

SERVES: 4

PREPARATION TIME: 15 minutes

COOKING TIME: 4 hours

INGREDIENTS:

Arrowroot starch ¼ cup

Black pepper ½ teaspoon

Chicken thighs 2 pounds (cut them into 1 inch pieces)

Coconut oil 1 tablespoon

Coconut aminos 3 tablespoons

Rice wine vinegar 2 tablespoons

Tomato paste or organic ketchup 2 tablespoons

Palm sugar ½-1 tablespoon

Garlic cloves, minced 2

Red pepper flakes ½ teaspoon

Raw cashews ½ cup

Extra equipment

Zip lock bag 1 large

METHOD:

1. Take a large zip lock bag and put black pepper and arrowroot starch into it.
2. Add pieces of chicken to the bag and seal. Toss it to thoroughly coat the meat.
3. Take a large skillet and melt coconut oil in it. Put chicken into the oil and cook for 5 minutes.
4. Put the chicken into the crockpot.
5. Mix red pepper flakes and coconut aminos in a small bowl. Sprinkle this mixture over the pieces of chicken. Toss again to

coat well.

6. Cover the crockpot with its lid and set it to low. Cook for 4 hours.
7. When the chicken is ready to serve, stir cashews into it.
8. Remove and place in a serving dish.

<u>Grass Fed Ribs</u>
METHOD:

This delicious umami flavored dish should be prepared way before you plan to eat it since the short ribs release a lot of fat into the gravy. If you do not want to consume that much fat, you can remove it when it hardens after you chill the ribs in the refrigerator.

SERVES: 6
PREPARATION TIME: 10 minutes
COOKING TIME: 9-11 hours
INGREDIENTS:

Grass fed ribs (short) with bone 6 pounds

Kosher salt as per taste

Ground pepper, fresh as per taste

Asian pear, cored, peeled, chopped 1 medium

Coconut aminos ½ cup

Garlic cloves, peeled and chopped 6

Scallions, chopped roughly 3

Ginger 2 inch piece

Red boat fish sauce 2 teaspoons

Coconut vinegar 1 tablespoon

Chicken broth 1 cup

Chopped cilantro, fresh 1 cup

<u>Mushroom Gravy Rump Roast</u>

You just need just 5 minutes to prepare this recipe before cooking. Come back from work and your amazing dinner will be waiting for you.

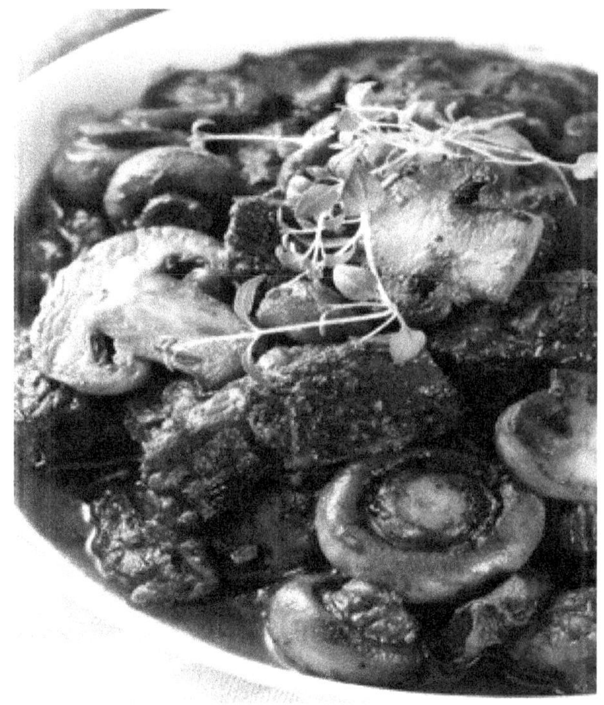

SERVES: 5-6
PREPARATION TIME: 5 minutes
COOKING TIME: 8 hours
INGREDIENTS:
Leftover beef roast 1-2 pounds
Chicken broth, low sodium, organic 3-4 cups
Roughly chopped onions 1-2 large
Peeled garlic cloves 5-6
Sliced mushrooms 1 container
Salt as per taste
Pepper as per taste
Garlic powder 1 teaspoon
Onion powder 1 teaspoon
Paprika ½ teaspoon
Coconut milk, full fat (canned) ½ cup

METHOD:

1. Place coconut milk, chicken broth, garlic, onions, mushrooms, and spices into the pot of your slow cooker. Stir well.
2. Make some space around the mixture of mushrooms and place little pieces of leftover beef roast into the mixture.
3. Cook on low for 7-8 hours. Set the cooker on high and cook for 4-6 hours further.
4. Remove to a serving bowl and you are ready to go!

<u>Apple Honey Ginger Shredded Pork</u>

Have you ever felt drunk after eating pork? Well, this pork might make you feel high since the taste is heavenly divine if you make it right. Invest in the time and you can thank us later.

SERVES: 6-8
PREPARATION TIME: 5 minutes
COOKING TIME: 8 hours
INGREDIENTS:
Shoulder roast of pork 2 pounds (you can also take any other roast)
Sliced, yellow onion 1 medium
Sliced and cored apples 2
Chicken broth, beef broth, or water 2/3 cup
Raw honey 1 tablespoon
Ginger, freshly grated 2 tablespoons
Cinnamon 1 teaspoon
Salt 1 teaspoon
Smoked paprika ½ teaspoon
Pepper ½ teaspoon
Garlic cloves, smashed 2
Bay leaf 1

METHOD:

1. Put chicken broth, beef broth or water into the pot of the slow cooker.
2. Add onions, and then pork. Put apples over the top.
3. Sprinkle spices in, pour in honey, and put bay leaf and garlic cloves into the pot.
4. Secure the cooker with a lid and set it on low. Cook for 8-10 hours.
5. Set on high and cook for 7-8 hours further.
6. Remove the meat onto a plate and use a fork to pull it apart.
7. Serve.

Moroccan Chicken with Slow Cooking

You might get bored with other slow cooked chicken dishes, but not with this one. This Moroccan chicken is a savory yet sweet dish bursting with flavor. It is full of Moroccan spices along with sweet apricots. You are going to truly appreciate the comfort of this exotic meal.

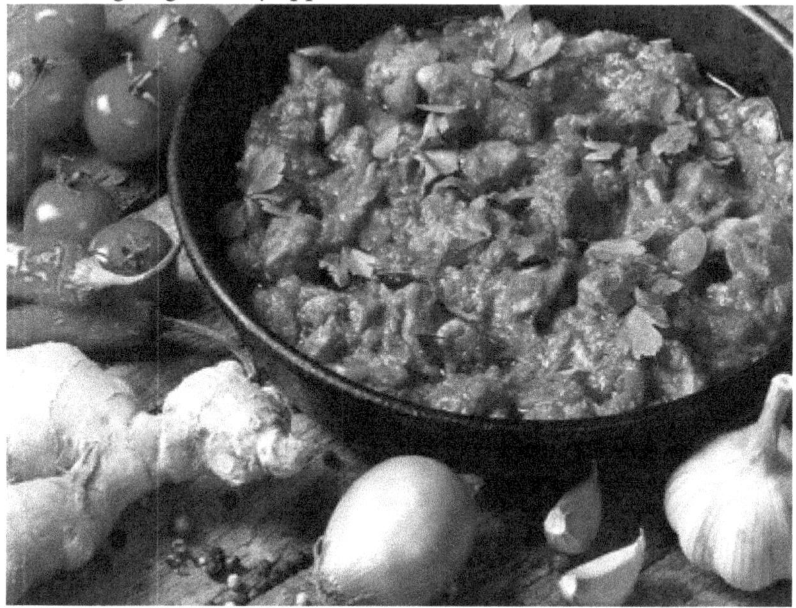

SERVES: 4-6
PREPARATION TIME: 15 minutes
COOKING TIME: 6 hours
INGREDIENTS:
Chicken drumsticks and thighs 2-3 pounds
Coconut oil or ghee 1 tablespoon
Onion, cut into vertical half rounds ½
Cumin powder 1 teaspoon
Turmeric powder 1 teaspoon
Coriander powder ½ teaspoon
Cinnamon powder ½ teaspoon
Cardamom powder ½ teaspoon
Cayenne powder ½ teaspoon (optional)

Minced fresh garlic 4 cloves
Fresh ginger, grated 1.5 tablespoons
Sea salt, unrefined 1.5 teaspoon
Bone broth 2 cups
Roughly chopped dry apricots 1 cup
Sweet potatoes, 1 inch pieces 2 cups
Fresh cilantro, chopped for garnish

METHOD:

1. Take a small bowl and put cumin, coriander, turmeric, garlic and cardamom into it. Stir well and keep aside.
2. Melt coconut oil or ghee in a large skillet over medium heat. Cook the chicken in this fat for 3 minutes. Flip over and cook for 3 minutes again. Do this step in batches if the skillet is small.
3. Transfer the chicken into the slow cooker.
4. Put onions into the skillet. Sauté for 4 minutes.
5. Add the spice mixture. Stir fry for 20 seconds so that the flavors come out well.
6. You can add more fat if you feel that the ingredients are sticking too much to the base of the skillet.
7. Add ginger, sea salt and bone broth to the skillet. Stir well and put the complete mixture of ingredients into the slow cooker.
8. Set the cooker on low and cook for 3 hours. Add sweet potatoes and dry apricots. Cover the cooker again and cook for 3 hours more.
9. Remove chicken to a serving dish and sprinkle chopped cilantro over for extra flavor and garnish. Serve.

<u>Curry Chicken</u>

The gravy of this chicken along with bell peppers tastes stronger than it looks. Indulge in the tender chicken breasts and thigh pieces and forget the worries of the day.

SERVES: 3-5
PREPARATION TIME: 10 minutes
COOKING TIME: 8 hours
INGREDIENTS:
Chicken breasts and thighs, skinless and boneless 2 pounds
Coconut milk ¾ cup
Tomato paste 2 tablespoons
Minced garlic 3 cloves
Ground ginger 1 tablespoon
Curry powder 4-6 tablespoons
Red and yellow bell peppers, cut into 1 inch pieces 2
Thinly sliced yellow onion 1
Salt as per taste
Pepper as per taste
Chicken broth 1 cup
METHOD:

1. Put coconut milk, garlic, ginger, tomato paste, curry powder, pepper and salt into the pot of your slow cooker. Stir well.
2. Add onions and bell peppers.
3. Put chicken into the pot and pour chicken broth over it.
4. Mix the ingredients well again.
5. Set the slow cooker at low and cook for 6-8 hours.
6. Set on high and cook for a further 4-5 hours.
7. Place in a serving bowl and serve hot.

Pork "Sausages"

Citrus and spices along with pork shoulder come together in this crockpot dish to give you a huge boost of flavor. Just bury everything a night before you plan to eat this meal and you will be welcomed with a tender pork meal.

SERVES: 4
PREPARATION TIME: 10 minutes
COOKING TIME: 8 hours
INGREDIENTS:

Onion 1 medium

Tomatoes, fire roasted 1x 15-ounce can

Annatto powder or paprika powder 2 tablespoons

Ground cumin 1 teaspoon

Black pepper 1 teaspoon

Salt 1 teaspoon

Nutmeg powder 1 pinch

Pork shoulder roast 5 pounds

Juiced orange 1

Apple cider vinegar ¼ cup

Salt 2 teaspoons

Coconut oil or ghee 1 tablespoon

METHOD:

1. Take a small bowl and mix cumin, annatto powder, salt (1 tsp), black pepper and nutmeg. Pour in a little water and stir to make a smooth paste.
2. Slice an onion.
3. Take a skillet and melt coconut oil or ghee over medium heat.
4. Sauté the onions until translucent and then add the canned fire roasted tomatoes. Let the tomatoes soften.
5. Prepare the pork: Remove any excess pieces of peripheral fat. The internal fat inside the meat will come out while cooking.
6. Cut out long slices of the roast approximately 1.5" wide. Sprinkle salt over them to season.
7. Take out your slow cooker. Pour orange juice in the pot along with apple cider vinegar.
8. Put in the spice paste and stir to blend them together.
9. Place the pork slices into the juice.
10. Top the pork with the onion and tomato mixture.
11. Set the cooker on low and cook for 8 hours.
12. When the pork is ready, the fat will start floating on the top. You can scoop it out. Alternatively, you can refrigerate the dish once cooled and the excess fat will harden on the top. You can then scoop it off easily.
13. Serve warm with onion rings and tomato wedges.

Crock Pot Balsamic Chicken with Sausage

If you are a fan of lots of seasonings, this balsamic chicken is just for you. After the meat is ready, just sprinkle some extra seasoning and you are ready to go with this marvellous dish.

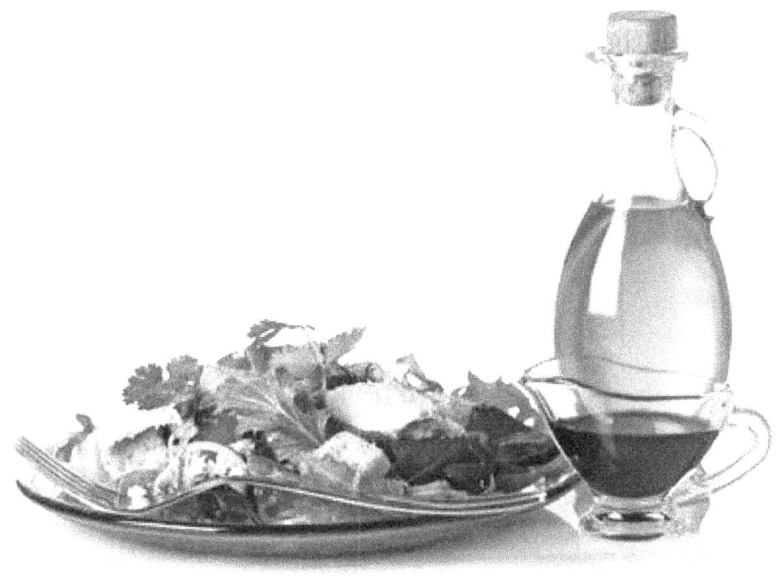

SERVES: 6-8

PREPARATION TIME: 10 minutes

COOKING TIME: 5 hours

INGREDIENTS:

Chicken breasts, boneless, skinless 4

Fresh sausage links, raw 6 (spicy or sweet or a combination)

Thinly sliced white onion 1

Chopped garlic 5-6 cloves

Olive oil, extra virgin 2 tablespoons

Italian seasoning 1 teaspoon

Garlic powder 1 teaspoon

Kosher salt 1 teaspoon
Diced tomatoes, organic 2 cans of 14.5 ounces
Tomato sauce 1 can of 15 ounces
Chicken stock or water 1 cup
Balsamic vinegar ½ cup
EXTRA SEASONINGS:
Italian seasoning 1 teaspoon
Kosher salt ½ teaspoon
Garlic powder ½ teaspoon

METHOD:

1. Lay the raw breasts at the base of the slow cooker. Drizzle 2 tablespoons olive oil over them.
2. Sprinkle over the Italian seasoning, salt and garlic powder.
3. Lay the raw sausages links on top of the chicken you've just seasoned.
4. Lay sliced onions and then chopped garlic over the sausages.
5. Put tomato sauce, diced tomatoes, balsamic vinegar and chicken stock into the slow cooker over the ingredients.
6. Top them with the extra seasonings mentioned in the ingredients. Do not stir. You will love the development of flavors in the end.
7. Secure the pot of slow cooker with its lid and set it to high. Cook for 5 hours.
8. Serve hot.

Yummy Beef Sandwiches

You must be wondering how you can eat sandwiches when you're not supposed to have bread. Do not worry. After all the slow cooker chicken, beef and pork; here's a change for you: some deliciously healthy sandwiches.

SERVES: 6-8
PREPARATION TIME: 20 minutes
COOKING TIME: 8 hours
INGREDIENTS:
Chuck roast, beef 2.5 pounds
Dried basil 1 teaspoon
Dried oregano 1 teaspoon
Crushed rosemary 1 teaspoon
Garlic powder 1 teaspoon
Onion powder 1 teaspoon
Salt ½ teaspoon
Black pepper ¼ teaspoon
Water ½ cup
Red wine vinegar 1 tablespoon
Dijon mustard 2 tablespoons
Portobello mushrooms, caps 6 large
Olive oil 1 tablespoon

METHOD:

1. Take a large skillet and pour 1 tablespoon of olive oil into it. Heat it over a medium high temperature.
2. Mix all the spices and coat the beef roast with them.
3. Sear the chuck roast on one side for at least 5 minutes in the skillet. Flip it over and cook for another 5 minutes.
4. Put it into the slow cooker and set the cooker to low. Cook for 8 hours.
5. Take out the meat and shred it using a fork.
6. If you see any fat in the slow cooker, scoop it out and discard it. Add Dijon mustard to the juices and stir.
7. Put the shredded beef back into the slow cooker.
8. Preheat the oven at a temperature of 450 degrees.
9. Take Portobello mushroom caps and season them with oil, pepper and salt.
10. Roast them in the oven for 10 minutes.
11. Use the mushrooms as buns and the shredded beef as a filling. Serve with roasted carrots, and cauliflower.

Slow Cooker Lasagna

This lasagna is an elaborate dish to prepare, but the time and effort are worth investing. You will not be able to forget the delicacy of this recipe for the next few weeks.

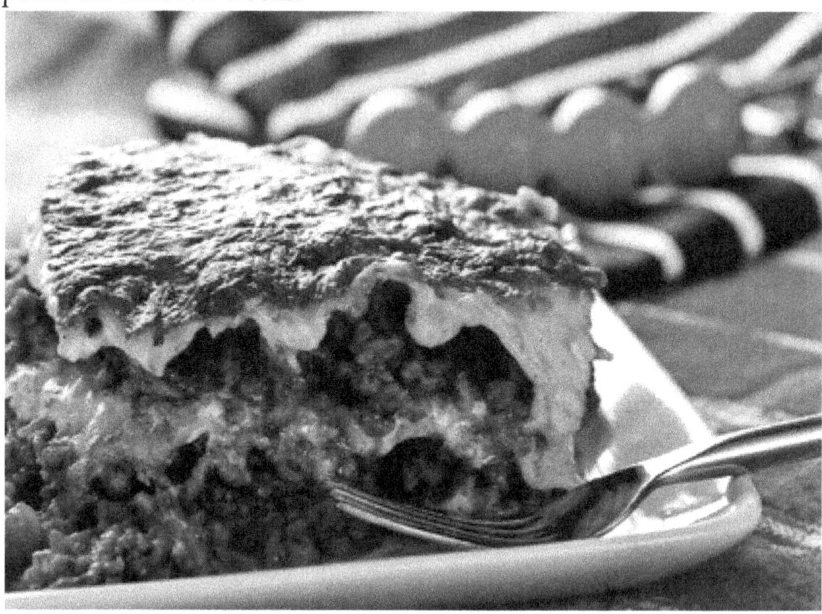

SERVES: 6-8
PREPARATION TIME: 20 minutes
COOKING TIME: 8 hours
INGREDIENTS (for marinara sauce):
Olive oil ¼ cup
Diced onion 1 small
Organic Salt 1 teaspoon
Minced garlic 1 teaspoon
Diced tomatoes 7 cups
Raw honey ½ tablespoon
INGREDIENTS (for meat filling):
Olive oil 1 tablespoon
Diced onion 1 small
Ground turkey 1 pound

Organic salt ½ teaspoon

Pepper ¼ teaspoon

Chopped basil leaves 18 large

INGREDIENTS (for cheese sauce):

Olive oil ½ tablespoon

Chopped onion ¼ small

Chopped yellow summer squash ½

Minced garlic ½ teaspoon

Organic salt ¼ teaspoon

Divided Coconut milk ½ cup

Egg 1

Thinly sliced zucchini (lengthwise) 4 medium (cut 6-7 slices of each zucchini)

METHOD (for marinara sauce):

1. Take a large saucepan. Heat olive oil over medium high temperature.
2. Add salt and onion. Sauté for 1-2 minutes.
3. Add garlic. Sauté for another 30 seconds.
4. Put in the honey and tomatoes and lower the heat to medium.
5. The sauce should cook for 20 minutes. When you see that it is not watery and has become thick, check the seasonings. Set aside.

METHOD (for meat filling):

1. Take a sauté pan and heat olive oil over medium high temperature.
2. Put ground turkey into the oil and break it apart using a spatula.
3. Let it cook for 2 minutes. Add onions, pepper and salt.
4. Let the ingredients cook until the turkey is thoroughly

cooked and small crumbles are formed. The onions will also become soft.

5. Remove the pan from the heat. Toss fresh leaves of basil into the pan. Stir.

METHOD (for cheese sauce):

1. Take a small saucepan and pour in the olive oil. Heat it over medium heat. Add yellow summer squash, chopped onions, garlic and salt. Sauté for 3-4 minutes. Let the onions become translucent, not brown.
2. Pour in ¼ cup coconut milk and bring it to the boil.
3. Simmer for 2 minutes or until more than half of the liquid has been absorbed.
4. Put the mixture into a blender jar. Pour the remaining ¼ cup coconut milk into the jar. Blend to make a smooth paste. Add egg and pulse again to blend all the ingredients well.

METHOD (for assembling lasagna):

1. Grease the inside of the slow cooker.
2. Pour ¾ cup of marinara sauce on the base of the slow cooker and spread it evenly.
3. Position about 5 slices of zucchini over the sauce.
4. Layer the zucchinis with cheese sauce using about ½ cup of it.
5. Sprinkle approximately ½ cup of the meat mixture over the cheese sauce.
6. Spread about ¾ cup of the remaining marinara sauce evenly over the meat mix.
7. You need to repeat this procedure to make at least 5 layers of cheese sauce, zucchinis, marinara and meat blend. The marinara sauce should come on top.
8. Cover the pot with its lid and set the cooker on high. Cook

for 1.5 hours.

9. Take off the lid.
10. Use a ladle or a turkey baster to take out the excess liquid that will have pooled in the slow cooker. Zucchinis release a lot of liquid.
11. Pour all the liquid in a frying pan and bring it to boil. Simmer for 4-6 minutes to make a creamy and thick sauce.
12. Pour this sauce over the lasagna in the slow cooker.
13. Serve hot.

<u>Crockpot Smashed Sweet Potato</u>

This is a very simple and fabulously nutritious recipe, which is mildly sweet as well. You can cook it for taking it along with you to a lunch at a friend's place.

SERVES: 4
PREPARATION TIME: 20 minutes
COOKING TIME: 4-5 hours
INGREDIENTS:
Sweet potatoes 2 pounds
Apple juice (without sugar) 1 cup
Ground cinnamon 1 tablespoon
Ground nutmeg 1 teaspoon
All spice mix ½ teaspoon
Ground cloves ¼ teaspoon
Pecans (optional)
Maple syrup or honey (optional, if you like it sweeter)
METHOD:

1. It is recommended to use a 3-4-quart slow cooker.
2. Peel the potatoes and cut them into slices of ½ inch each.
3. Put the potatoes in the slow cooker.
4. Pour in ½ cup of the apple juice along with the spices.
5. Cook for 4-5 hours on low until the potatoes become tender.
6. When the potatoes are cooked thoroughly, add the remaining ½ cup of apple juice.
7. Blend the mixture using a hand blender.
8. Add more seasoning of nutmeg and cinnamon as you like.
9. Remove the potatoes and place them in a serving bowl. Top with pecans.

<u>Stuffed Bell Peppers</u>

The Italian flavor of these bell peppers stuffed with sausages and cauliflower is absolutely delicious, and they are simple to make. You can have this dish for lunch and feel satiated for the rest of the day.

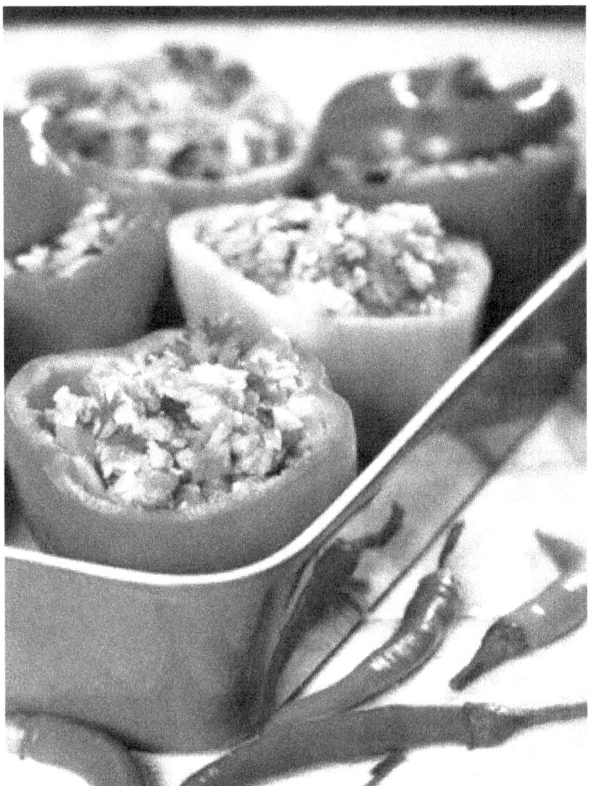

SERVES: 4
PREPARATION TIME: 10 minutes
COOKING TIME: 6 hours
INGREDIENTS:
Italian hot sausage (ground) 1 pound
Bell peppers 2 red, 2 green, 1 yellow
Cauliflower ½ head
Tomato paste 1 can of 8 ounces
White onion, diced 1 small

Minced garlic ½ head
Dried basil 2 teaspoons
Dried oregano 2 teaspoons
Dried thyme 2 teaspoons
METHOD:

1. Cut off the top portion of the bell peppers. Discard the seeds but keep the tops.
2. Chop the cauliflower into the consistency of rice.
3. Add garlic, onion and herbs to the cauliflower and mix.
4. Heat a skillet on high and light brown the sausage.
5. Add the sausage and tomato paste into the cauliflower mix and combine them using your hands.
6. Fill up the bell peppers with this mixture and place them into the slow cooker. Cover the peppers with their tops.
7. If any mixture remains behind in the bowl, stuff it between the bell peppers.
8. Set the cooker on low and cook for 6 hours.
9. Take out and serve.

Gingerbread Apple Pudding Cake

This is an enchanting dessert. It will get baked like a simple cake, but will create its own sauce on the bottom like that of a pudding, and all this will happen in the slow cooker!

SERVES: 4

PREPARATION TIME: 10 minutes
COOKING TIME: 2.5 hours
INGREDIENTS:
Apples (peeled and cut into cubes of ½ inches) 3 medium
All-purpose flour 1.25 cups
Granulated sugar ¼ cup
Baking soda 1 teaspoon
Salt ¼ teaspoon
Ground ginger ¾ teaspoon
Ground cinnamon ½ teaspoon
Ground nutmeg ¼ teaspoon
Water ½ cup
Molasses 1/3 cup
Vegetable oil 2 tablespoons
Brown sugar ½ cup
Apple cider 1.25 cups
Butter
2 tablespoons
METHOD:

1. Spray the slow cooker using cooking spray.
2. Position the apples evenly on the base.
3. Take a bowl and put in the flour, baking soda, sugar, ginger, cinnamon, salt, and nutmeg. Mix them well.

4. Take another bowl and mix the molasses, oil and water. Put it into the dry ingredients and mix well.
5. Spread this mixture over the apples. Sprinkle some brown sugar over the top as well.
6. Take a microwavable cup. Microwave butter and apple cider for 2-3 minutes to boil the mixture. Pour the liquid slowly and evenly into the slow cooker over the batter. Do not mix.
7. Cook for 2.5 hours on high. Turn off the slow cooker and let it stand for 15 minutes.
8. Serve.

Choco-Peanut Nuggets

With the simplest of ingredients, this dessert is going to take your heart away. The sweet nuggets are good when you are on the go.

SERVES: 4

PREPARATION TIME: 10 minutes

COOKING TIME: 2.5 hours

INGREDIENTS:

Candy coating (Vanilla flavored) 16 ounces

Candy coating (chocolate flavored) 16 ounces

Salted peanuts, dry roasted 16 ounces

Unsalted peanuts, dry roasted 16 ounces

METHOD:

1. Take a 4 quart slow cooker and put candy coatings in the pot.
2. Cook them on low for 2-3 hours. Stir occasionally till they melt completely.
3. Put peanuts into the mixture and coat them thoroughly.
4. Spread the mixture on parchment paper to cool and harden.
5. It will cool down within an hour. Break into pieces and store in an airtight container.

Conclusion

Slow cooker recipes sound difficult but they are much easier than they appear. After reading so many crockpot recipes, you should be feeling more positive about this technique. There are various pieces of equipment associated with slow cooking. You will have read about them in the initial part of this book. The purpose of writing *Paleo Diet Lovers: The Ultimate Paleo Crock-Pot Cookbook for Busy People* is to help you get acquainted with this method and various recipes which you can experiment with.

The major advantage associated with this method is that you can try out various ingredients with each recipe and the outcome will be positive in each case. But, you must do so with proper knowledge of each ingredient. The cooking time for all foods is different. If you follow these timings, they come out beautifully.

Also, you can experiment with different types of equipment for slow cooking. Each of them has a specific taste associated with them. For example, chicken cooked in slow cooker will be juicy but will take more time. The same chicken recipe cooked in a pressure cooker will be denser and will take much less time. There is no harm in testing different types of apparatus. You can use whichever of them suits you the best.

There is no limit to learning with cooking. The same ingredients can be cooked in at least ten different ways. Just be bold and keep going with your new adventure.

Good luck!

Gluten Free Paleo Cookies and Desserts. Sweet Tooth Cravings Sorted.

By: *Emily Simmons*

Table of Contents

<u>Banana bacon cookies</u>
<u>Macadamia nut cookies</u>
<u>Orange blossom cookies</u>
<u>Sunflower cookies</u>
<u>Lazy espresso cookies</u>
<u>Avocado double chocolate cookies</u>
<u>Sandwich cookies</u>
<u>Conclusion</u>

Introduction

When we say "Paleo diet", we are referring to following a diet chart which uses ingredients from the Stone Age. But there was not a trace of sugar or dessert in that age. Our ancestors did not even know about it. But what are we to do when we see so many delicious desserts all around us? Our sweet tooth starts craving sweets even more when we look at or smell delicious sweets and foods. However, no need to worry. Even in the Paleo diet, we have a lot of options to make and bake cookies, cakes and desserts using healthy ingredients.

Gluten Free Paleo Cookies offers numerous options for making cookies and other desserts. If you are a chocolate fan, you will find the initial few recipes filled with dark chocolate and cacao. However, if you want a change from chocolate, you can switch to blueberries, lemon, maple syrup, bacon and many other things to satiate your taste buds. You seem to never get enough of unhealthy desserts, but are constantly left craving more. But Paleo desserts are fully satisfying. They satisfy your sweet tooth in the best possible way and do not make you crave sweetness all day long. Moreover, you can indulge in these sweets as much as you want without any guilt because they are made up of absolutely natural ingredients.

People these days are more concerned about their health than ever before. Thus, they prefer remaining hungry to eating unhealthily. But it is neither good for the body nor practical to go without desserts when all your friends are savoring delicacies of cakes and pastries after a dinner. Thus, it has become more of a necessity to have healthy options for main courses as well as desserts; not only to satisfy your cravings, but also to maintain your social life.

Open this book and explore a world of beautiful, healthy cookies. Enjoy!

How to Handle your Sweet Tooth Cravings.

It is really next to impossible to escape your cravings for sweet treats. However, we do not mean to discourage you- not at all. Even when you cut down on the usual culprits- candy, simple carbohydrates and desserts, there are many places where sugar can sneak into your diet. Even the healthiest of foods contain a lot of sugar. For instance, 8 ounces of a regular smoothie contains 28 grams of sugar. This is very close to the 26 grams of sugar in a similar quantity of cola. Amazed, aren't you?

Don't worry. We all get cravings for one thing or the other every now and then. Not cheating on your Paleo diet requires a huge amount of will-power and most of us, of course, do not have it. The solution is to know how and where to cheat. When we know the right substitutes, we can cheat the cheating as well!

Change what cheating means to you

The best way to reduce the effects of cheating is to change the definition of cheating for you. It means that you have to find out about healthier cheat foods for when you have cravings. When you consume these healthier "cheat foods", you can get "off the menu" and still remain healthy.

List your favorite sweet foods from your previous lifestyle. Typically, they are some of these: Nutella, Red Bull, Snickers, peanut butter, ice-creams, doughnuts, etc. Now, you just have to substitute these foods with Paleo alternatives like: dark chocolate, bacon, avocado, raspberries, banana, whipped cream coffee, whipped cream with berries, frozen fruit smoothies, red wine, and almonds.

The most important benefit of these Paleo cheat foods is that most of these are self-limiting foods. You may recall that you could not stop yourself from eating a whole box of vanilla sundae. But you cannot eat a complete bar of very dark chocolate or cacao. You feel satiated early, and when you consume less, you are also consuming fewer calories.

What You Can do to Control Yourself From Eating Non-Paleo Desserts

Everyone needs a break from all those "healthy" foods. You might want to allow yourself to deviate from that healthy path now and again. But no one wants to go back 4 weeks just because of a single craving. Go through the following tips to readjust your cravings.

If there is cheat food in your home, you will eat it

Avoid buying foods that you don't want to eat yourself. Buying ice-cream for the guests who are due to come next week is just an excuse. You know in your heart that you are going to eat it in the next two days. Do not buy it before you need it.

Eat cheat foods that satisfy your cravings

When you eat ice-cream, you feel guilty and unsatisfied afterwards. So, what is the use of eating any such food which does not satisfy your cravings? Instead, eat foods which will satisfy you and not make you feel terrible afterwards.

Think of the prize of being on Paleo

When you remember your goal of a better physique, better moods and good health, you will not feel guilty or deprived while you are on a Paleo diet. If you constantly think of foods that you cannot eat, you will feel negative and more vulnerable to give into temptations of unhealthy foods. If you think positively about the abundance of foods that you *can* eat, you will not feel deprived.

How to Beat Your Cravings Without Willpower

Controlling your cravings needs much more than just willpower. You can save the willpower for emergency situations, when you just have to control your cravings. Use these methods to tackle your cravings on a day-to-day basis:

You must prevent your cravings

You might be wondering how that's possible. You must eat when you feel hungry. If your stomach calls for food, it's hunger, not craving. Feed your body with quality protein and fat. You will not have as many cravings if your stomach is satisfied. Do not deprive yourself of carbohydrates and fats. When you do, you crave them even more. Eat Paleo friendly carbs and fats.

Distract yourself

You can distract yourself if you feel the craving for anything unhealthy. Try these methods:

Read a novel.

Watch your favorite show on TV.

Open an album of old photos.

Do yoga.

Paint, knit, crochet, sew or do anything to keep yourself busy.

Take a siesta.

Stay happy

You might just be feeling down and thinking of it as cravings. You can do something else to cheer yourself up instead of eating fast food. Try these ideas:

Visit an interesting place.

Take time out just for yourself, even if it is very unproductive. You do not have to answer to anyone for taking a break.

Surprise a friend by randomly showing up.

Do anything that you think is fun.

Do not feel embarrassed about the craving.

Do not let the craving make you feel guilty forever. If you think of it as just a passing phase which everyone experiences, it will become more manageable. Acknowledge it and let it pass.

Replace your cravings

We have already spoken about this. You can substitute your cheat foods with healthier Paleo foods such as Paleo crackers, Paleo cakes, Paleo cookies, Paleo pizza, Paleo ice-cream etc.

Go to a healthy place

It becomes easier to stop craving pizza if you are not forced to smell it. You get the point, right? Remove yourself physically from the place where you feel more cravings, instead of staying there and trying to fight them.

Paleo Cookies Recipes
Paleo Samoas

These Paleo samoas are just awesome. Serve them chilled and your family will ask for them over and over again.

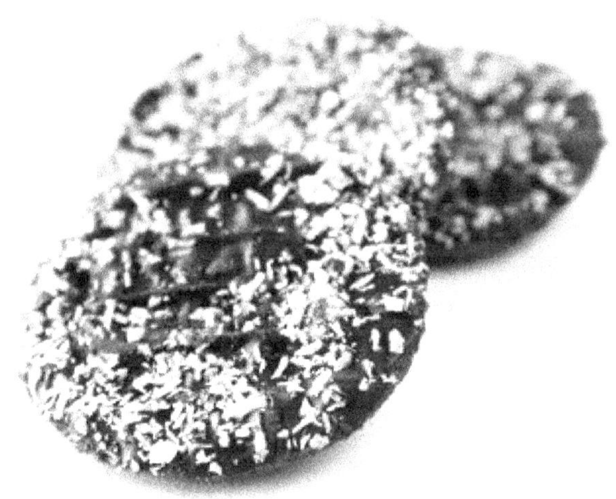

SERVES: 5-6
PREPARATION TIME: 1 hour
INGREDIENTS:
Shortbread cookies:
Almond flour 2 cups
Coconut flour ¼ cup
Coconut sugar ¼ cup
Butter (at room temperature) 10 tablespoons
Vanilla extract 2 teaspoons
Baking soda ¼ teaspoons
Honey caramel:
Raw honey ½ cup

Nut butter (unsalted- cashew, pecan or almond) 2 tablespoons
Vanilla extract 1 teaspoon
Chocolate drizzle:
Chopped cacao butter ½ cup
Cacao powder 5 tablespoons
Raw honey 2 tablespoons
Unsweetened coconut flakes ¼ cup
METHOD (for cookies):

1. Preheat the oven to a temperature of 350 degrees. Line your baking dish with unbleached parchment paper.

2. Mix all dry ingredients for cookies- almond flour, coconut flour, coconut sugar and baking soda. Add vanilla and softened butter. Blend in the butter using a fork.

3. As you keep on blending, the mixture will form into a ball of dough. Wrap it in parchment paper. Refrigerate it for 1 hour.

4. Place the refrigerated dough between two sheets of unbleached parchment paper.

5. Roll it into ¼- ½ inch thick layer.

6. Take a 2.5 inch cookie cutter, and cut out cookies. Roll the dough again and repeat the procedure until you finish the dough.

7. Place the cookies on the baking dish and cook for 12 minutes in the oven or until they become golden brown.

8. Remove the cookies onto a cooling rack. Let cool completely.

METHOD (for chocolate drizzle and honey caramel):

1. Heat a small saucepan over medium heat and add honey. Let it heat for 3-5 minutes and keep stirring occasionally. When you see small bubbles rising from the pan, lower the heat.

2. Take it off the heat and mix in vanilla and nut butter. The caramel will be in a liquid state when you mix the ingredients

and will firm up gradually while cooling down.

3. Heat another small saucepan over low heat. Melt honey, cacao powder and cacao butter. Cook for 3-5 minutes or until a smooth paste is made. Keep aside.

METHOD (for assembling cookies):

1. Place the cookies on the baking sheet lined with parchment paper and frost them with caramel. Drizzle chocolate on top of the cookies and sprinkle with coconut flakes.
2. Refrigerate the cookies and serve chilled.

Bacon Maple Chocolate Cookies

Bacon never fails to please in the Paleo diet. Apart from being added to other gluten free recipes, bacon pieces taste wonderful in these chocolate cookies as well.

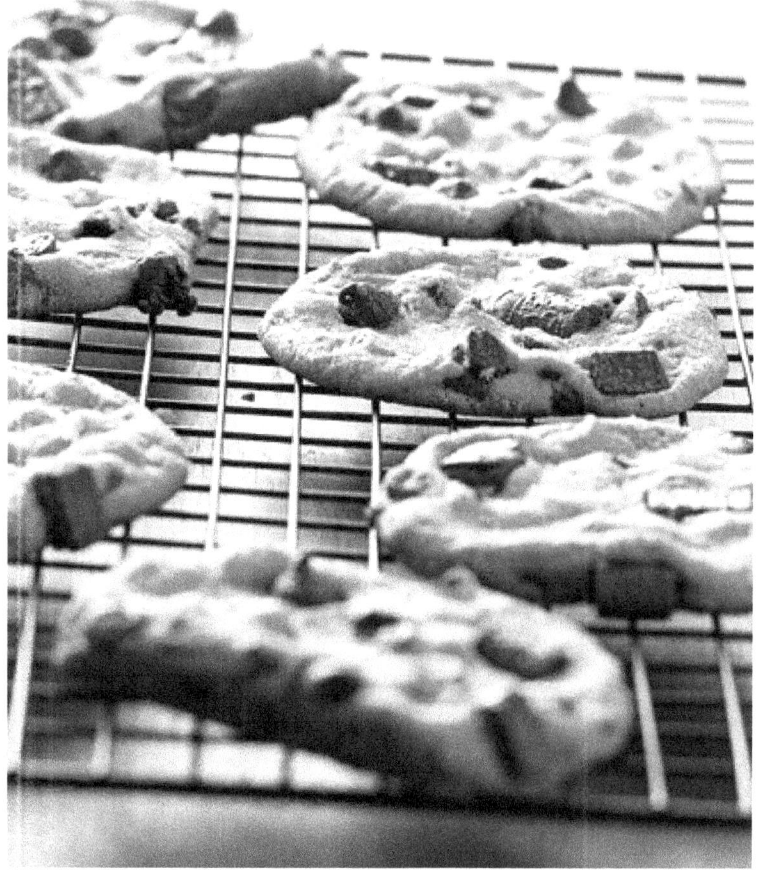

SERVES: 5-6

    PREPARATION TIME: 1 hour

    INGREDIENTS:

Bacon 4 slices

Bacon fat 2-3 tablespoons

Almond flour 1 cup
Chocolate chips ½ cup
Eggs 2
Maple syrup 3 tablespoons
Vanilla extract 1 teaspoon
METHOD:

1. Preheat the oven to a temperature of 350 degrees Fahrenheit.
2. Take a pan and heat it over medium heat. Cook bacon slices until the fat is released. You can cook some extra slices too for munching on later.
3. While the bacon is cooking, combine all other ingredients (except bacon fat and bacon) and mix properly.
4. When the slices of bacon are cooked, chop them into pieces of ¼– ½ inches. Slightly larger pieces give a better texture to the cookies. Break the pieces using clean hands only.
5. Add the pieces of bacon into the bowl containing other ingredients and add bacon fat. Combine well.
6. Line a baking sheet with aluminum foil and scoop out the mixture in equal measures over the baking sheet. You can use a measuring spoon for this purpose.
7. Put it into the oven and cook for 10 minutes or until you see that the edges have become golden brown. The center will become firm when thoroughly cooked.
8. Serve hot or cooled, as you prefer.

Chocolate Chip Blueberry Cookies

Blueberries have tremendous health benefits. They not only keep your bones healthy, but also help in digestion and to fight wrinkles. So, all the pretty ladies out there! Gobble down these healthy Paleo blueberry cookies without any guilt and reap the benefits.

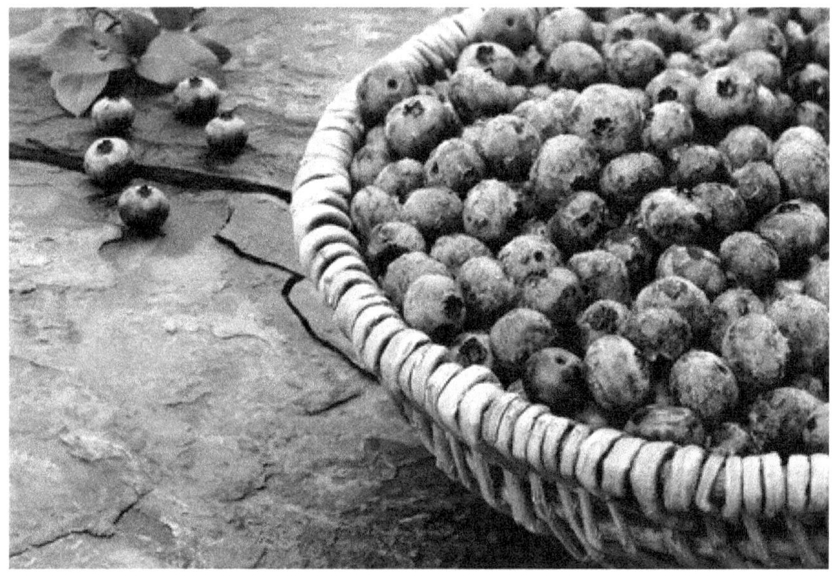

SERVES: 3-4

PREPARATION TIME: 35 minutes

INGREDIENTS:

Blueberries 2 cups

Walnuts 2 cups

Walnut oil/ almond oil/ coconut oil 2 tablespoons

Almond flour 1.5 cup

Chocolate chips (dark) 1/3 cup

Maple syrup 3 tablespoons

Whisked egg 1 medium
Cinnamon 1 tablespoon
Vanilla extract 1 teaspoon
Baking soda ¼ teaspoon
Salt a pinch
Coconut crystals for topping

METHOD:

1. Preheat the oven to a temperature of 400 degrees Fahrenheit.
2. Take a baking sheet and line it with parchment paper.
3. Take a medium saucepan and put blueberries in it over low-medium heat. Let them cook for 10 minutes. Keep stirring frequently.
4. While the blueberries are cooking, add walnuts to the jar of a food processor. Process until the walnuts turn into chunky butter.
5. Now, add blueberries to the jar with walnut butter. Process to blend them together.
6. Take out the batter and place in a large bowl. Put in the rest of the ingredients. Combine them well.
7. Using an ice cream scoop or a tablespoon, take out 2 scoops of batter for each cookie on the baking sheet. Your batter should make 14-15 cookies.
8. Put the baking tray in the oven and bake for 20-23 minutes.
9. Take the cookies out of the oven and let cool. The cookies may be sticky. If so, use a plastic spatula to remove them when they cool down.
10. Serve.

<u>Chocolate Chip Sweet Potato Cookies</u>

Enjoy your sweet potato cookies with a cup of coffee and indulge in the heavenly taste of these unforgettable cookies.

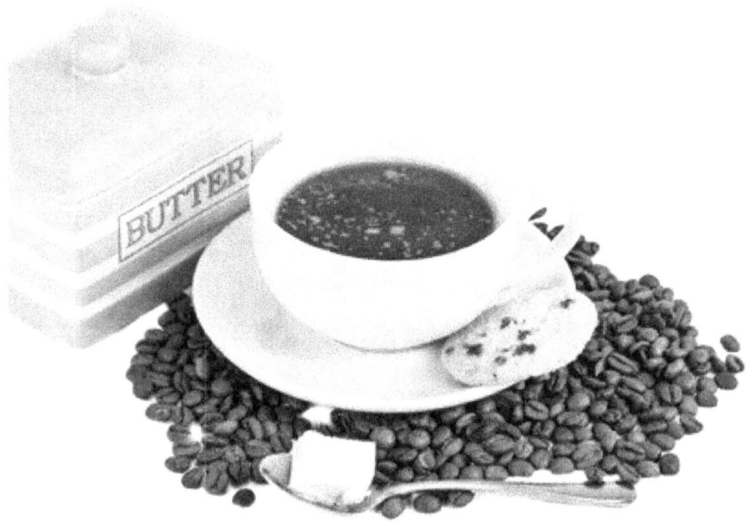

SERVES: 3-4

PREPARATION TIME: 50 minutes

INGREDIENTS:

Sweet potato 1 small

Almond butter (smooth) ½ cup

Whisked egg 1 medium

Honey 1 tablespoon

Vanilla extract 1 teaspoon

Vanilla protein powder 35 grams (1 scoop)

Cinnamon 1/8 teaspoon

Salt a pinch
Chocolate chips ½ cup
METHOD:

1. Preheat the oven to a temperature of 400 degrees Fahrenheit.
2. Poke holes in the potato and place it in the oven to be baked for 35-40 minutes. The potato should become completely soft.
3. Take the potato out and let it cool. Reduce the oven temperature to 350 degrees.
4. Peel the potato and put it in a bowl. Mash it using a fork.
5. Add egg, almond butter, vanilla extract and honey. Combine the ingredients well.
6. Add cinnamon powder, salt, and protein powder to the same bowl. Mix them well.
7. Add chocolate chips and fold them in well.
8. Take a baking sheet and line it with parchment paper.
9. Take tablespoons of the batter and place them on the baking sheet. 12-13 cookies can be made with this amount of batter.
10. Place the baking sheet in the oven and cook for 10-12 minutes. Take out the cookies and let cool. Serve. You can also sprinkle some chocolate chips on top of the cookies immediately after you take them out of the oven.

Chocolate Chunk Cookies

Very easy to make and quick to cook- these cookies are just the thing when your sweet tooth wants something urgently! Cook them in a jiffy and enjoy!

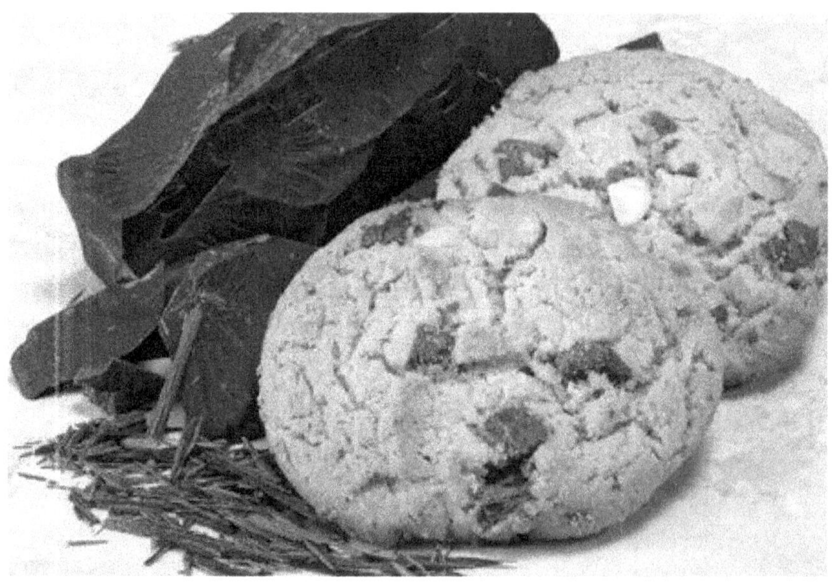

SERVES: 3

PREPARATION TIME: 20 minutes

INGREDIENTS:

Sunflower seed butter (chunky) 1 cup

Honey 1/3 cup

Egg 1

Vanilla 1 teaspoon

Cinnamon 1 tablespoon

Baking powder ½ teaspoon

Baking soda ½ teaspoon

Salt as per taste

Chopped walnuts ½ cup

Chocolate chunks ½ cup

METHOD:

1. Preheat the oven to a temperature of 350 degrees Fahrenheit.
2. Take a medium sized bowl and put in all the ingredients. Mix well.
3. Take a baking dish and line it with parchment paper.
4. Take a large spoon put scoops of the batter onto the baking dish. Leave plenty of space between each scoop.
5. Put the dish into the preheated oven and cook for 12-15 minutes.
6. Take the dish out and serve cookies.

<u>Chocolate Cranberry Cookies</u>

Again, you have a recipe that's easy to make and just delicious. Cranberry cookies. They look lovely, and they taste amazing as well.

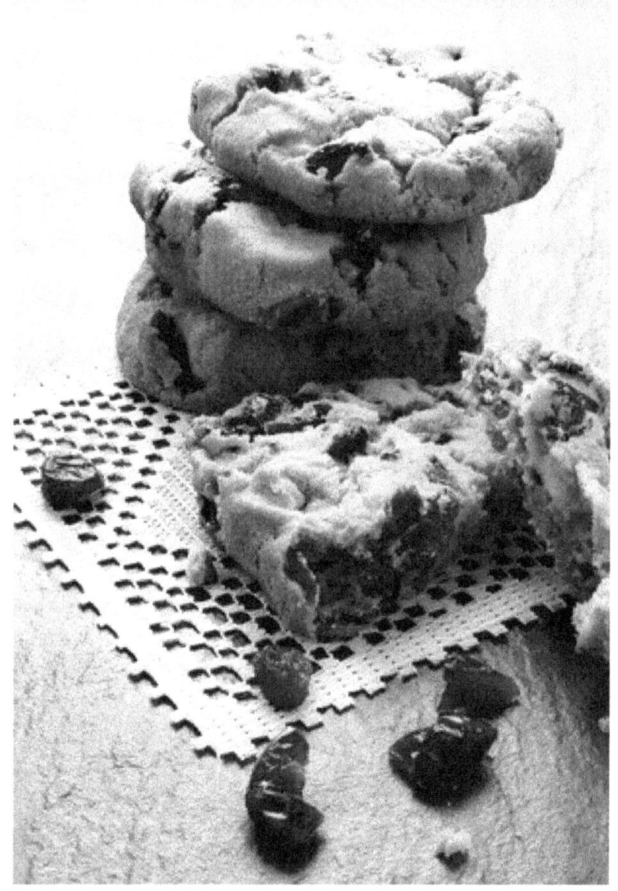

SERVES: 4

PREPARATION TIME: 20 minutes

INGREDIENTS:

Ground flaxseed 1 tablespoon

Water 3 tablespoons or

Egg 1 large

Roasted almond butter ½ cup
Coconut sugar ½ cup
Vanilla extract ½ teaspoon
Baking soda ¼ teaspoon
Salt 1/8 teaspoon
Chopped cranberries (frozen) ¼ cup
Chocolate chips ¼ cup
METHOD:

1. Preheat the oven to a temperature of 350 degrees Fahrenheit.
2. Take a cookie sheet and line it with parchment paper. Alternatively, you can also grease it using cooking spray.
3. Put flaxseed in a small bowl and whisk them using water to form "flax egg". It will form into a gel after five minutes. You can also use egg in place of water.
4. Take another bowl and mix coconut sugar, almond butter, baking soda, vanilla extract and salt. Combine the ingredients well.
5. Put chocolate chips and chopped cranberries in the mixture. Add the flax egg as well. Combine well.
6. When the dough is properly formed, make balls of equal size and place them on the baking sheet. You can moist your hands with water if you feel that the dough is too sticky or moist.
7. Place the baking sheet into the oven and cook for 13 minutes. Let them cool on the baking dish before placing them on a cooling rack.
8. When the cookies reach room temperature, serve.

Chocolate Chip Double Almond Cookies

Flax egg has tremendous health benefits. You can add it to any cookie recipe you like to obtain its goodness.

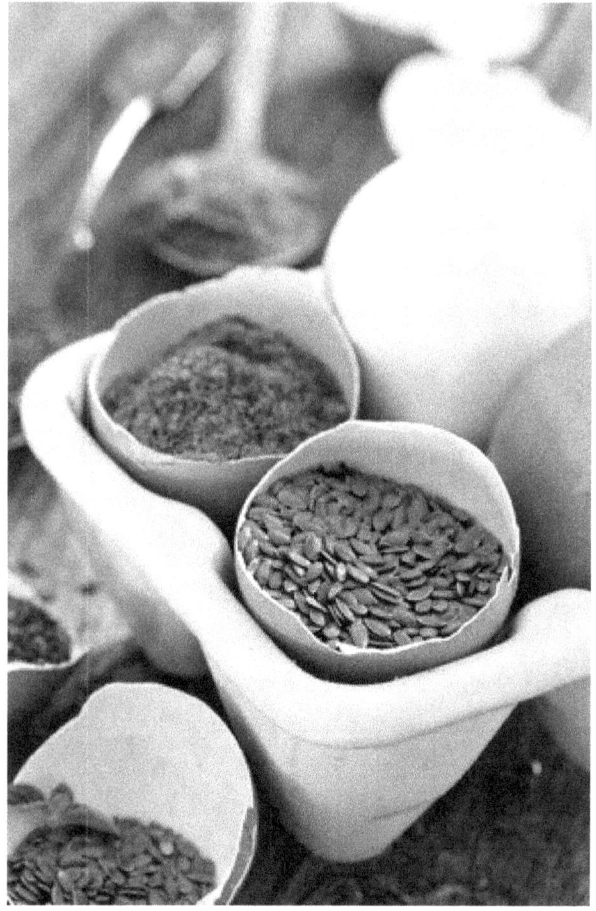

SERVES: 15

PREPARATION TIME: 1 hour

INGREDIENTS:

Ground flaxseeds 1 tablespoon

Water 3 tablespoons

Coconut sugar 1 cup

Almond butter (unsalted, roasted) 1 cup

Vanilla extract 1 teaspoon

Espresso powder 1 teaspoon
Salt ½ teaspoon
Coconut flour ¼ cup
Baking powder 1 teaspoon
Dark chocolate chips ½ cup
METHOD:

1. Preheat the oven to a temperature of 350 degrees Fahrenheit.
2. Put flaxseeds in a small bowl and whisk them using water to form "flax egg". It will form into a gel after five minutes. You can also use egg in place of water.
3. Take a large bowl and put coconut sugar, flax egg, almond butter, espresso powder, vanilla extract, and salt. Combine well.
4. Add baking powder and coconut flour gradually to form a soft dough.
5. Add chocolate chips.
6. Make balls of the size of a heaping tablespoon.
7. Place the balls on a baking sheet. Flatten them using your palm.
8. Use plastic wrap to cover the baking tray. Keep it in the refrigerator for 60 minutes.
9. Take out the baking dish and remove the plastic sheet.
10. Put the dish into the oven and cook for 7-8 minutes. The cookies should become golden brown.
11. Let them cool on the baking tray before you transfer them to the cooling rack.

Chocolate and Bacon Cookies

Feel free to experiment with this lovely recipe. Substitute some ingredients here and there and you will still end up with delicious cookies.

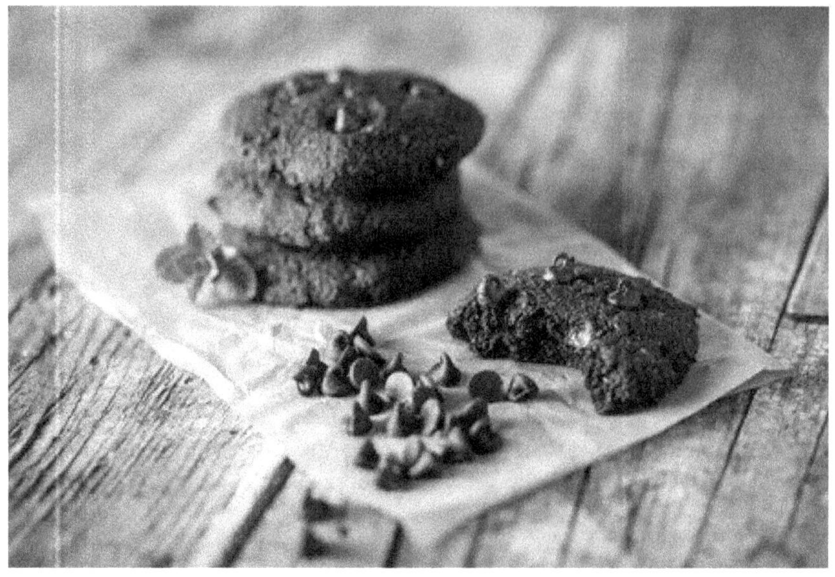

SERVES: 2-3

PREPARATION TIME: 20-25 minutes

INGREDIENTS:

Almond flour 1 cup

Salt 1/8 teaspoon

Baking soda 1/8 teaspoon

Coconut oil (melted) 3 tablespoons

Honey 2 tablespoons

Vanilla extract 1 teaspoon

Coconut or almond milk 1 teaspoon

Dark chocolate (chopped) ¼ cup

Bacon (cooked, crumbled) 2-3 tablespoons/ 2 slices

METHOD:

1. Preheat the oven to a temperature of 350 degrees Fahrenheit.
2. Take a cookie sheet and line it with parchment paper.
3. Take a bowl and combine salt, baking soda and almond flour.

Mix well.

4. Put all the wet ingredients in a separate bowl and whisk them together.

5. Add bacon and chocolate to the bowl of dry ingredients. Pour wet ingredients over them. Combine them well using a spatula.

6. Wet your hands and make balls of about 1.5 heaped tablespoons.

7. Place the balls on the baking sheet and press them using your palm.

8. Put the baking sheet into the preheated oven and cook for 10-12 minutes.

9. Let them cool for 3-5 minutes.

10. While the cookies are still soft, sprinkle with a little sea salt.

11. Place the cookies on the wire rack.

Cookie Dough Paleo Bites

What else do you need from a cookie recipe when it does not need baking? You save all the effort of baking and still get to enjoy the treat.

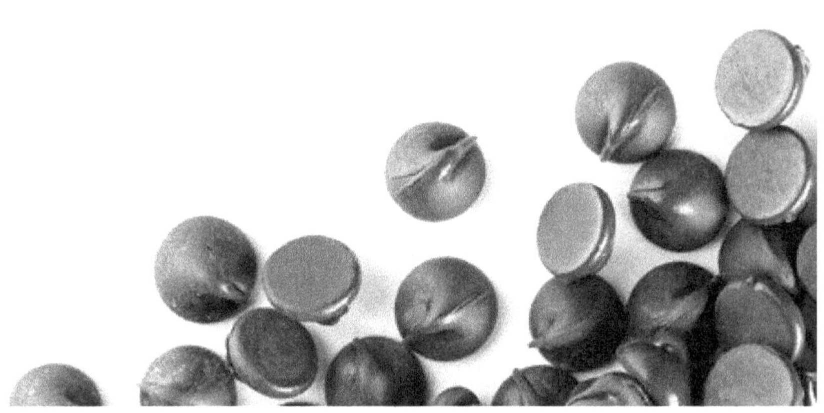

SERVES: 2-3

PREPARATION TIME: 20 minutes

INGREDIENTS:

Melted coconut oil 3 tablespoons

Full fat coconut milk 1.5 tablespoons

Vanilla extract ¾ tablespoons

Raw honey 2 tablespoons

Almond flour (blanched) ¾ cup

Chocolate chips 3 tablespoons

Chocolate chips 1 tablespoon (for drizzling)

METHOD:

1. Take a cookie sheet and line it with parchment paper.

2. Take a medium sized bowl and put coconut milk, coconut oil, honey and vanilla.
3. Use a rubber spatula to mix the almond flour into the ingredients in the bowl. Combine them well. Do not over mix the batter or it may become oily.
4. Add chocolate chips and fold them in the batter.
5. Keep the dough in the refrigerator for 30 minutes.
6. Roll the dough into tablespoon-sized balls. Place them on the baking sheet.
7. Melt some chocolate chips using double boiler method over simmering water.
8. Drizzle melted chocolate over the cookies.
9. Refrigerate for a while and then serve.

Paleo Oreos

Now you do not have to stop your kids from eating the whole packet of Oreos. You can hand over a bunch of these homemade Paleo Oreos to them! They will be eating something healthier and enjoying it as well.

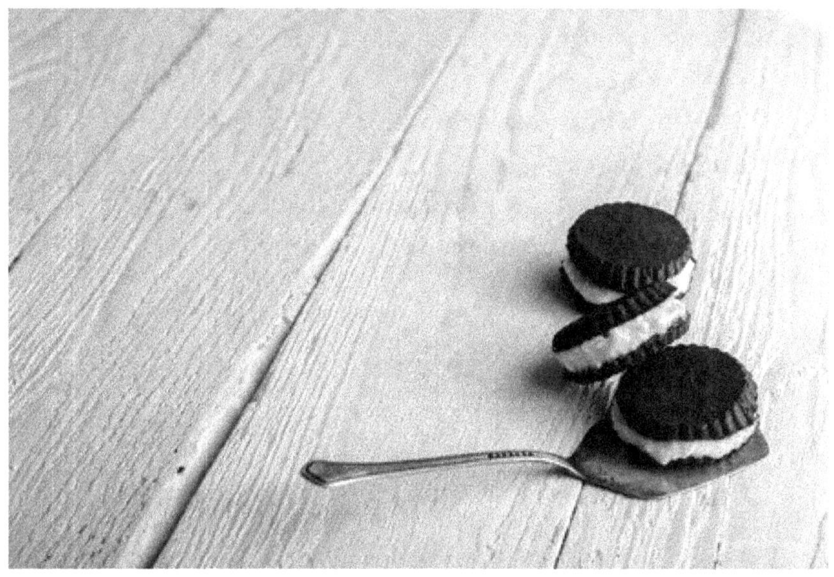

SERVES: 2-3

PREPARATION TIME: 20 minutes

INGREDIENTS (for cookies):

Almond flour (blanched) ½ cup

Arrowroot powder ¼ cup

Cacao powder (raw) ¼ cup

Butter (at room temperature) 4 tablespoons

Full fat canned coconut milk 1 tablespoon

Vanilla extract ½ teaspoon

Raw honey 2 tablespoon

INGREDIENTS (for buttercream filling):

Melted coconut butter 3 tablespoons
Vanilla extract ½ teaspoon
Water 2 tablespoons
Raw honey 1 tablespoon
METHOD (for cookies):

1. Mix arrowroot powder, cacao powder and almond flour in a medium bowl.
2. Add wet ingredients to this mixture. Combine them well and put it in the refrigerator for 15 minutes.
3. Take another bowl and mix coconut milk, butter, raw honey and vanilla extract.
4. Take the bowl out of the refrigerator and make a ball of the dough. Roll the ball between 2 parchment paper sheets. The thickness of the dough should be around 1/8 inch.
5. Remove the top sheet of the parchment paper. Transfer the lower sheet along with dough onto a baking sheet.
6. Cut out 2-inch cookies using a cookie cutter and remove the remaining dough. It can be used for making more cookies.
7. Bake the cookies in the oven at 350 degrees Fahrenheit for 10-11 minutes. They should become light golden in color.
8. Take the baking sheet out and let the cookies cool. After a few minutes, place them on a cooling rack.

METHOD (for buttercream filling):

1. Mix the ingredients of the buttercream and combine them well in the small jar of your mixer.
2. Put about 1 teaspoon of buttercream in the center of one cookie. Place another cookie on top and press them together gently.
3. Serve when they cool down.
4. Store the remaining cookies at room temperature.

Chocolate Chunk Sunbutter Cookies

Butter made from sunflower seeds is perfect for satiating your taste buds as well as for reaping health benefits. It's used in this recipe to make some amazing cookies.

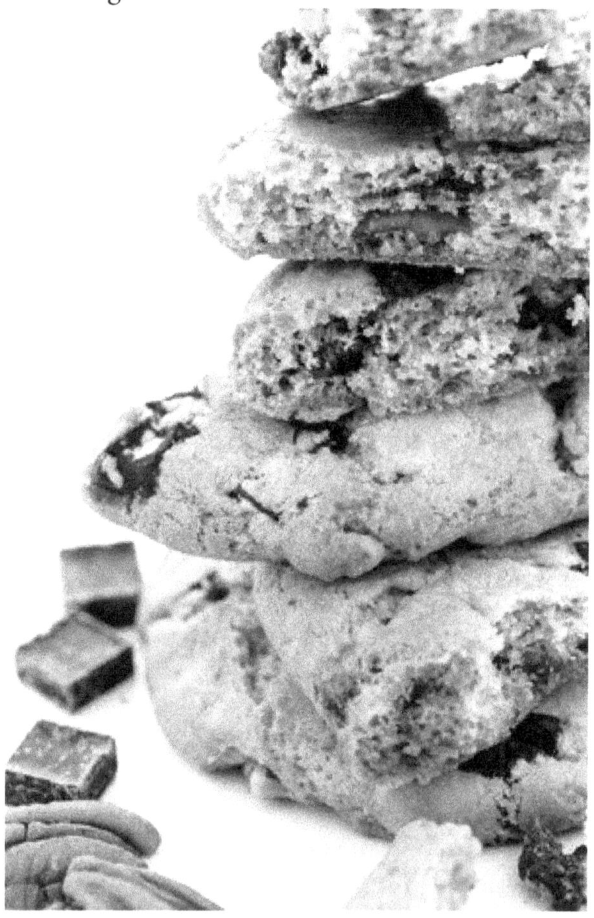

SERVES: 6

PREPARATION TIME: ½ hour

INGREDIENTS:

Sunflower seed butter ½ cup

Almond butter ½ cup

Beaten egg 1

Vanilla extract 2 teaspoon

Maple syrup 1/3 cup

Cinnamon ½ teaspoon

Baking soda ½ teaspoon

Baking powder ½ teaspoon

Salt ¼ teaspoon

Chopped dark chocolate 1 cup

Sea salt 1 teaspoon

METHOD:

1. You can make sunflower butter from the seeds yourself if you do not want to buy it. Put 2 cups sunflower seeds in a jar of your food processor. Process it until you get a creamy and smooth butter.

2. Preheat the oven to a temperature of 350 degrees Fahrenheit.

3. Take a large bowl and mix all the ingredients, keeping aside chocolate chunks. Mix the ingredients well until they are combined to form a batter.

4. Fold in the chocolate chunks.

5. Take a baking sheet and line it with parchment paper. Scoop out the batter on the sheet and make six cookies.

6. You can sprinkle sea salt over the cookies if you like.

7. Put the baking sheet into the oven and cook for about 18-20 minutes. They should become golden brown.

8. Let them cool and then serve.

<u>Pumpkin Cake Chocolate Cook-ies</u>

You might have become bored with all these similar-looking cookie recipes. Here, we have a break in the monotony for you. These pumpkin cookies are a combination of cake and cookies. They are softer on the top and crisp at the bottom. Enjoy!

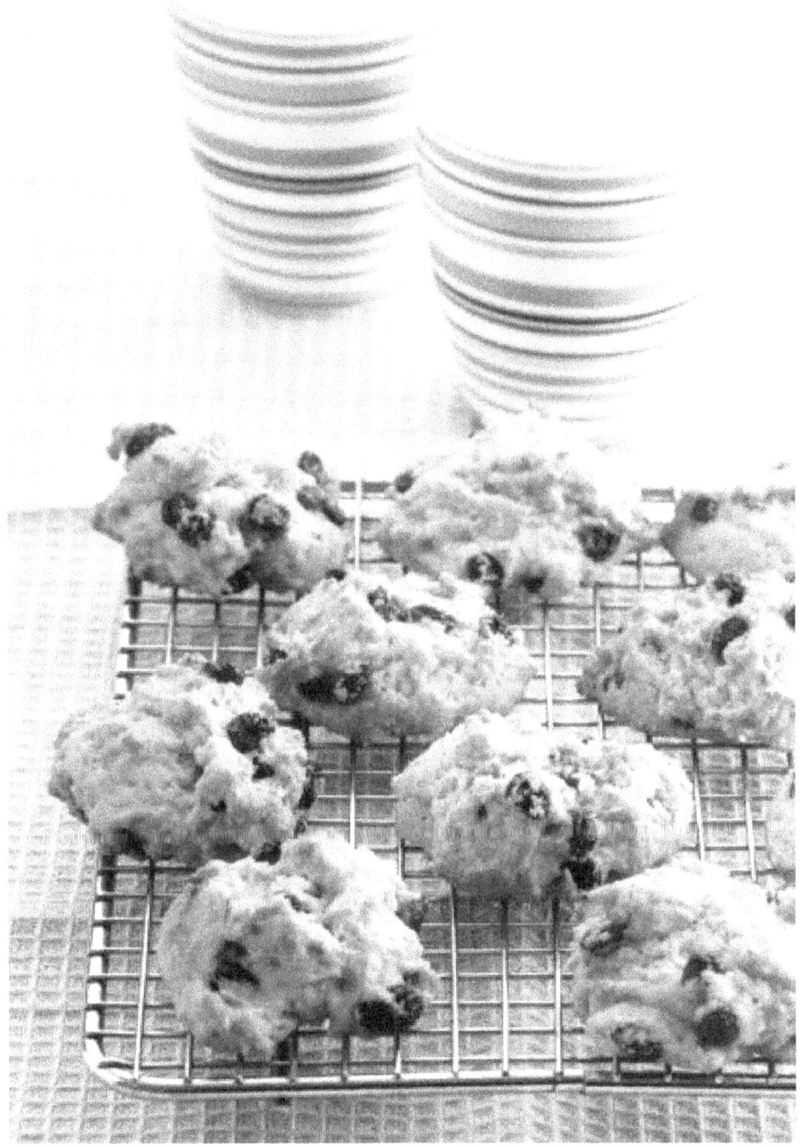

SERVES: 20

PREPARATION TIME: 20 minutes

INGREDIENTS:

Pumpkin/sweet potato/banana puree ¾ cups

Coconut flour ½ cup
Melted coconut oil ½ cup
Eggs 6
Vanilla extract 2 teaspoons
Honey ¼ cup
Cinnamon 1 teaspoon
Nutmeg 1 teaspoon
Allspice mix 1 teaspoon
Baking powder ½ teaspoon
Chocolate chips 1 cup

METHOD:

1. Preheat the oven to a temperature of 350 degrees Fahrenheit.
2. Take the jar of your electric mixer and put in coconut oil, pumpkin, honey, eggs and vanilla. Process to combine the ingredients.
3. In a bowl, sieve cinnamon powder, nutmeg, coconut flour, baking powder and allspice mix.
4. Add this flour to the mixer jar and process to combine them. There should be no clumps in the batter.
5. Add chocolate chips and fold them in the batter,
6. Take a baking sheet and line it with parchment paper.
7. Scoop out the dough around the size of a large tablespoon on the baking sheet.
8. Put the sheet in the oven to cook for 11-12 minutes. The bottoms should be cooked in this time.
9. You will find these cookies are not like normal ones. The upper crust should be softer and the bottom harder.
10. Take them out of the oven and let cool slightly.
11. Serve warm.
12. You can store them in an airtight jar for 3 days.

Grain Free Chocolate Bars

The goodness of walnuts along with the taste of chocolate is a perfect combination. Just a little innovation in the shape of cakes, cookies and bars can add a new touch of fun to your breakfast.

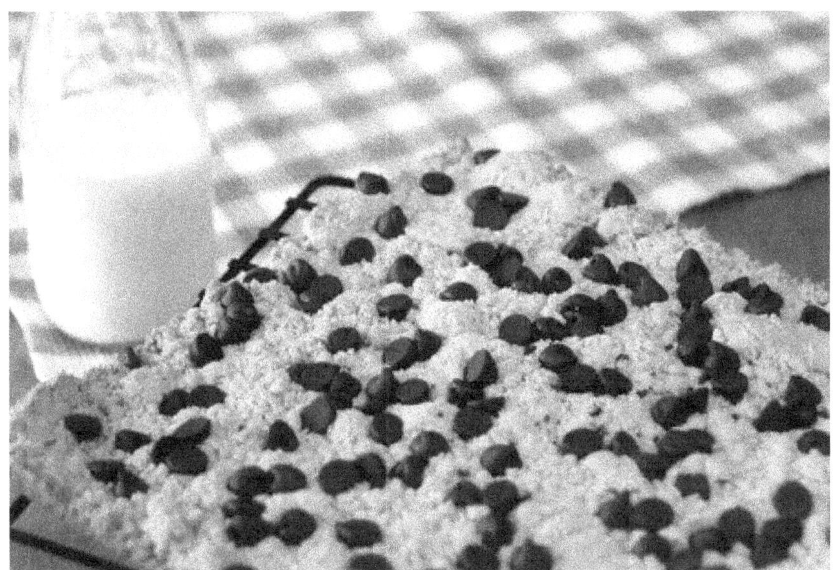

SERVES: 4-5

PREPARATION TIME: 40-50 minutes

INGREDIENTS:

Almond flour (blanched) 2.5 cups

Baking soda 1 teaspoon

Sea salt ½ teaspoon

Honey 1/3 cup

Brown eggs 2 large

Melted coconut oil ¼ cup

Vanilla extract 2 teaspoons

Almond milk 1 tablespoon

Chocolate chips (semi-sweet) ¾ cup

Walnuts ¼ cup
METHOD:

1. Preheat the oven to a temperature of 350 degrees Fahrenheit.
2. Take an 8" baking pan (square) and grease its sides and bottom with coconut oil.
3. Take a large bowl and put all dry ingredients in it.
4. Take another small bowl and whisk all wet ingredients together with a hand whisk.
5. Now pour the wet mixture into the large bowl containing dry ingredients. Combine them using the hand blender.
6. Add chocolate chips and fold them in the batter.
7. Pour the batter into the greased baking pan. Spread it evenly using a spatula.
8. Put it in the oven for 20-25 minutes until the top crust is cooked and golden brown.
9. Take out of the oven and let cool for 10-15 minutes.
10. Cut the cake carefully into bars.
11. Store the bars in an airtight container in the refrigerator.
12. Microwave to warm up before serving.

<u>Vegan Chocolate Cookies</u>

These light and crumbly cookies have yummy chocolate chunks inside them. If you enjoy larger bits of chocolate in your sweets, this recipe is for you.

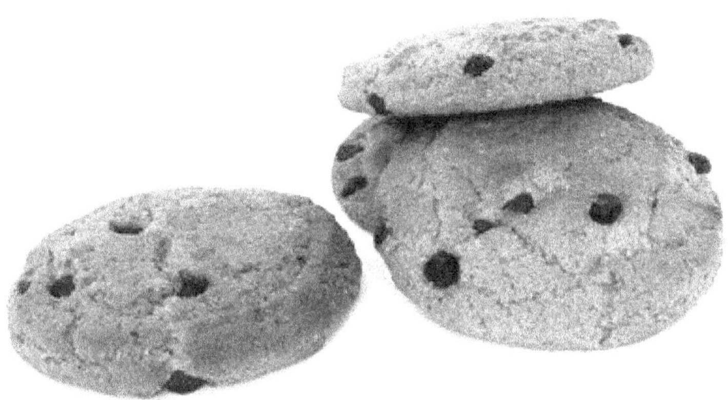

SERVES: 4-5

PREPARATION TIME: 30-40 minutes

INGREDIENTS:

Almond meal 1 cup

Sea salt ¼ teaspoon

Baking soda 1/8 teaspoon

Cinnamon ¼ teaspoon

Melted butter or coconut oil 3 tablespoons

Maple syrup or honey 2 tablespoons

Vanilla extract 1.5 teaspoons

Water 0.5-1 teaspoon

Dark chocolate, chopped/ chocolate chips 3-4 tablespoons

METHOD:

1. Preheat the oven to a temperature of 350 degrees Fahrenheit.
2. Take a medium sized bowl and put in salt, almond meal, cinnamon and baking soda. Mix them well.
3. Take another bowl and mix maple syrup/ honey, coconut oil and vanilla extract.
4. Pour these wet ingredients into the other bowl. Add enough water to bind the ingredients together.
5. Add chopped chocolate pieces and stir in.
6. Take a baking sheet and line it with parchment paper.
7. Scoop out 2 tablespoonfuls of batter for each cookie onto the baking sheet.
8. Bake the cookies for 10-12 minutes until the edges become golden.
9. Take out the baking sheet and let the cookies cool.
10. Take them out and enjoy!

Gluten Free Cookies

A ball of chocolate-packed cookie, when it crumbles in your mouth, does not leave you any option but to think of heaven. Indulge in the crime of gobbling these cookies down. Shhhhhh! Do not tell your mom!

SERVES: 15

PREPARATION TIME: 25-30 minutes

INGREDIENTS:

Softened coconut butter ¾ cup

Brown sugar ¾ cup

Coconut oil 3 tablespoons

Large eggs 2

Baking soda ½ teaspoon

Kosher salt ½ teaspoon

Almond flour 3 cups

Chocolate chips 6 ounces

METHOD:

1. Preheat the oven to a temperature of 350 degrees Fahrenheit.
2. Soften the coconut butter. Combine it with coconut oil and brown sugar. Beat the ingredients for 2-3 minutes in a mixer with paddle attachment.
3. Add an egg to the mixture. When the egg is fully mixed, add the other egg. Now, add kosher salt and baking soda.
4. Pulse the mixture on a medium-low speed. Gradually add almond flour to avoid making lumps. Mix them well.
5. Add chocolate chips and fold them completely.
6. Make balls of about 2 tablespoons of the dough using your hands. Put the balls on a baking sheet. You can flatten them if you like.
7. Bake them for 10-11 minutes until the balls become light

brown on the top.

8. Take the cookies out of the oven and let cool. Serve after 5-10 minutes.

Cut Out Grain Free Cookies

The icing on top just provides the finishing touch to these delicious cookies.

SERVES: 10-12

PREPARATION TIME: 1 hour

INGREDIENTS (for cookies):

Almond flour, blanched 2 cups

Sea salt ¼ teaspoon

Baking soda ¼ teaspoon

Coconut oil, virgin, melted ¼ cup

Honey ¼ cup

Vanilla extract 1 tablespoon

INGREDIENTS (for icing):

Chilled coconut milk, full fat 1 can

Honey 1 tablespoon

METHOD (for cookies):

1. Preheat the oven to a temperature of 350 degrees Fahrenheit.
2. Take a medium sized bowl and mix baking soda, salt and almond flour.
3. Take a small bowl and whisk honey, coconut oil, vanilla extract, and honey together.
4. Add the whisked mixture to the bowl of flour and blend together until you get a smooth paste.
5. Take a large baking sheet and line it with parchment paper.
6. Roll the dough between two parchment paper sheets. The thickness should be about ¼ inches. Freeze the dough for 5 minutes after rolling out. This makes it easy to cut.
7. Cut out the cookies using cookie cutters and place them on the baking sheet.
8. Freeze the cut out cookies for 5 minutes so that they can hold

their shape during baking.

9. Bake them for 10-12 minutes. The cookies will become golden brown at the edges.

10. Take them out and let cool for a few minutes, then place on cooling racks.

11. Repeat the procedure for the remaining dough.

METHOD (for icing):

1. Scoop out coconut cream from the can into a small bowl. Keep the remaining milk for making smoothies later.

2. Pour honey over coconut cream and whisk until smooth. Transfer the mixture into a piping bag. Pipe the cream on the cookies after they have cooled down. Keep the remaining cream in an airtight jar and store in a refrigerator.

Paleo Macadamia Cookies

You might have become bored of eating dark chocolate. Here we have macadamia nut cookies for you to give to your taste buds a change.

SERVES: 4-5

PREPARATION TIME: 45 minutes

INGREDIENTS:

Macadamia nuts, raw, whole ¾ cups

Almond flour 1 cup

Desiccated coconut, unsweetened 1 cup

Ground ginger 1 teaspoon

Honey ¼ cup

Melted Coconut oil ¼ cup

Baking soda ½ teaspoon

Water, divided 2 tablespoons

METHOD:

1. Preheat the oven to a temperature of 320 degrees Fahrenheit.
2. Spread macadamia nuts on the baking sheet. Bake for 5-7 minutes and roast them slightly. Chop the nuts roughly when they're slightly cool.
3. Reduce the heat of the oven to 250 degrees Fahrenheit.
4. Take a large bowl and mix desiccated coconut, almond flour, ginger and macadamia nuts.
5. Take a saucepan and pour in coconut oil and honey. Melt them gently.
6. Take a small bowl and mix water (1 tablespoon), and baking soda. Add this mixture to the coconut oil mixture.
7. When you see the mixture frothing up, take the saucepan off from the heat. Pour the ingredients onto the wet ingredients. Add 1 more tablespoon of water into this mixture and combine well.

8. Take a baking sheet and line it with parchment paper.
9. Take an ice cream scoop and make 12 cookies or more if you have more batter.
10. Place the cookies on the baking sheet. Flatten the cookies using the back side of the scoop.
11. Put the sheet into the oven and bake for 22-25 minutes. The cookies will become golden brown.
12. Take out the cookies and let them cool. Serve.

Brownie Bites

Baking is eliminated, but taste is not! These cookie balls are just so easy to make and taste equally as good. These little cookie balls are bound to be a hit with the whole family. Serve them as after dinner truffles if you like, too.

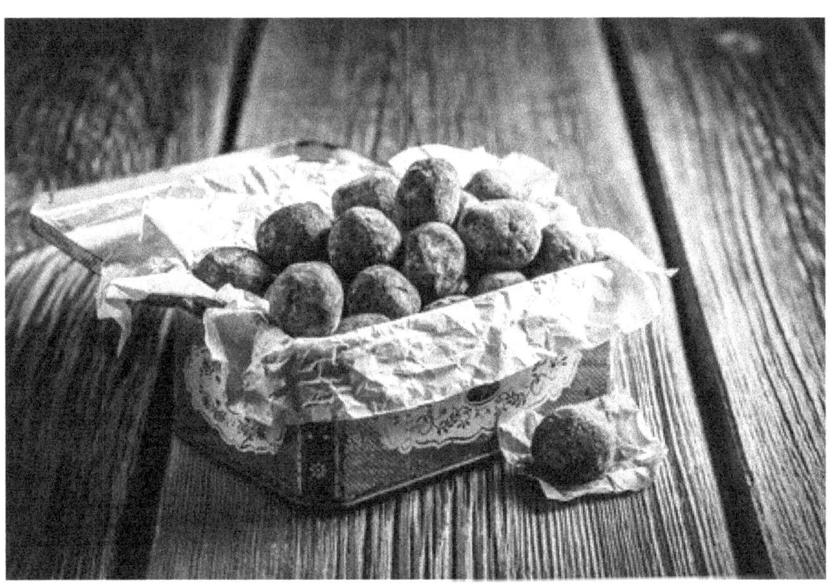

SERVES: 4-5

PREPARATION TIME: 45 minutes

INGREDIENTS:

Walnut halves 1.5 cups

Cocoa powder ¼ cup

Vanilla extract 1 teaspoon

Sea salt ¼ teaspoon

Pitted soft dates 10

Water 1 tablespoon

Cocoa powder to coat

METHOD:

1. Take the jar of food processor with "S" blade. Grind the walnut halves into a smooth meal.
2. Put the remaining ingredients in the jar. Process until a sticky dough is formed. The dough should be uniform in consistency.
3. Take a baking sheet and line it with parchment paper.
4. Scoop out heaped teaspoons of dough.
5. Roll the dough into balls, using your hands. Roll the cookies in cocoa powder.
6. Refrigerate the cookie balls and serve chilled.

Banana Bread Chocolate Cookies

SERVES: 4-5
PREPARATION TIME: 20-25 minutes
INGREDIENTS:
Eggs 2
Softened Butter 1.5 tablespoons
Mashed banana ½ cup
Almond milk ¼ cup
Honey ¼ cup
Vanilla 1 teaspoon
Coconut flour ½ cup
Cinnamon ½ tablespoon
Baking powder 1 teaspoon
Sea salt 1/8 teaspoon
Dark chocolate chips ½ cup
METHOD:

1. Preheat the oven to a temperature of 350 degrees Fahrenheit.
2. Mix butter, eggs, banana, honey, vanilla and almond milk in a bowl.
3. Take another bowl and mix cinnamon, coconut flour, salt and baking powder. Add this mixture to the other bowl. Combine all the ingredients well.
4. Put in chocolate chips and fold them in well.
5. Take a baking sheet and line it with parchment paper.
6. Take out a spoonful of batter for each cookie, place on the baking sheet, and flatten them with the back side of the spoon.
7. Put the baking sheet into the oven and cook for 18-20 minutes.

8. Remove from oven and let cool for 5 minutes. Transfer the banana cookies onto a cooling rack.
9. Serve.

Sugar Lemon Cookies

You can experiment with the look and feel of these wonderful lemon cookies. Eat them as single cookies or join two together with lemon curd- just as you like. They will taste awesome either way.

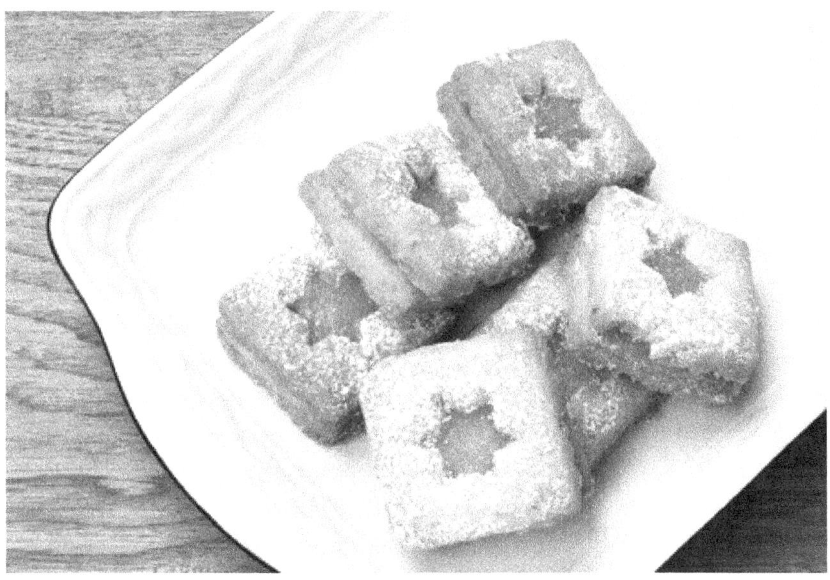

SERVES: 3-4

PREPARATION TIME: 25 minutes

INGREDIENTS (for cookies):

Ground almonds 2 cups

Arrowroot powder 1 tablespoon

Baking soda ¼ teaspoon

Salt ¼ teaspoon

Melted coconut oil ¼ cup

Maple syrup ¼ cup

Vanilla extract 1 tablespoon

Lemon zest 1 small lemon

INGREDIENTS (for lemon curd):

Water 60 milliliters
Arrowroot powder 3 tablespoons
Maple syrup 60 milliliters
Lemon zest and juice 1 small lemon
Turmeric or yellow edible color ½ teaspoon

METHOD (for cookies):

1. Put arrowroot powder and ground almonds in the food processor. Process to make powdery flour. Sieve the flour into a medium bowl. Discard the lumps.
2. Pour maple syrup, coconut oil, lemon zest and vanilla extract into the food processor. Pulse until the ingredients are combined well.
3. Return the sifted flour to the food processor. Pulse until a smooth dough is formed.
4. Pack the dough between two sheets of cling film. Roll it till about ½ cm thick. Chill in the refrigerator for 20 minutes.
5. Preheat the oven to a temperature of 338 degrees Fahrenheit and line a baking sheet with parchment paper.
6. Remove the dough from the refrigerator and roll it between two sheets of parchment paper.
7. Cut out cookies using cookie cutters. Cut half of the cookies full in shape and half of them with the center cut out.
8. Place them on the baking tray and cook for 8-10 minutes. Do not let the cookies brown excessively.
9. Let them cool on a wire rack before joining together with lemon curd.

METHOD (for lemon curd):

1. Mix arrowroot powder and water in a saucepan. Dissolve the powder properly in the water.
2. Heat it over medium heat and bring the mixture to boil. The

mixture will thicken gradually while you stir.

3. Drizzle maple syrup in gradually and cook on medium heat for a minute.
4. Take the saucepan off the heat and pour the mixture in a plastic bowl. Put in lemon zest and juice and mix. Add turmeric or yellow color and combine the ingredients.
5. Let it cool, and whisk before serving. When the spread is ready, spread on the whole cookies and top with the ones that are cut out in the center. You can refrigerate the lemon curd in the refrigerator for 3 days.

Thumbprint Blueberry Cookies

The jelly-like texture of the filling in these thumbprint blueberry cookies is just so good that you'll want to have more than two at a time! Blueberries are good for you, so that's alright.

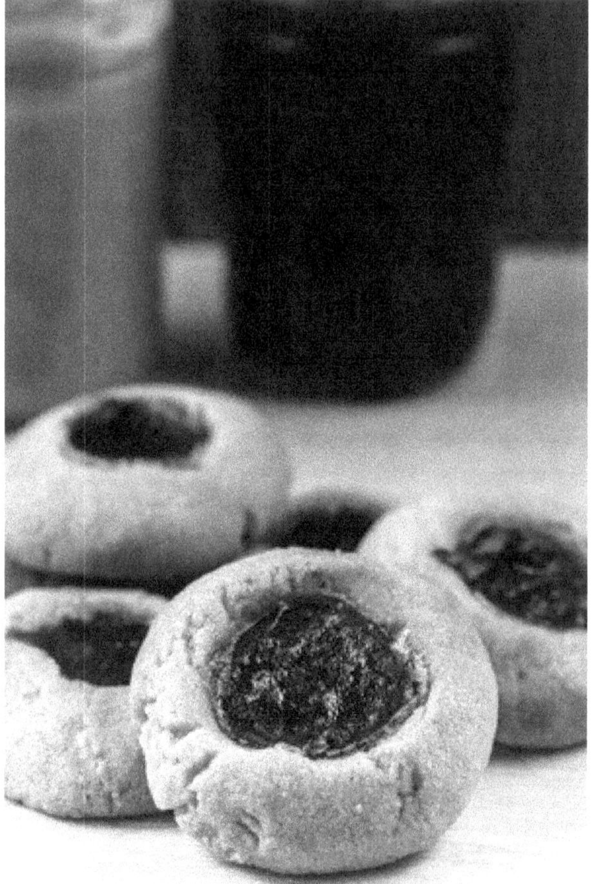

SERVES: 10

PREPARATION TIME: 35 minutes

INGREDIENTS (for filling):

Blueberries 2 cups

Maple syrup 1 tablespoon

Water ¼ cup

Lemon juice ¼ cup

Nutmeg ½ teaspoon

Cinnamon 1 teaspoon

Arrowroot powder 1-2 tablespoon

INGREDIENTS (for cookies):

Almond flour, blanched 2 cups

Arrowroot powder 1 cup

Arrowroot powder 1/2 cup (dusting)

Salt 1 teaspoon

Vanilla extract 1 teaspoon

Maple syrup 1/3 cup

Melted coconut oil, organic ¼ cup

METHOD (for filling):

1. To prepare filling, heat a saucepan over medium heat and put in maple syrup, blueberries, lemon juice, water, cinnamon and nutmeg.
2. Stir continuously and let the mixture boil. You can a use a wooden spatula to mash the berries.
3. When you see the liquid reducing, turn down the heat and put in the arrowroot powder. Let the filling thicken, stirring continuously.
4. Remove the saucepan from the heat and let the mixture cool. You can add more blueberries to the filling mixture at this stage if you want.

METHOD (for cookies):

1. Preheat the oven to a temperature of 350 degrees Fahrenheit.
2. Take a large bowl and mix arrowroot powder, salt and almond flour.
3. Add vanilla extract, coconut oil and maple syrup. Combine all

the ingredients well and make a dough ball. You can make the dough using your hands as well.

4. Take a baking sheet and line it with parchment paper.
5. Make small balls of the dough and place on the baking sheet. Use all the dough. You can use arrowroot powder for dusting if you find the dough is too sticky.
6. Press your thumb in the middle of the rolled cookies to make a well.
7. Put about a tablespoon of blueberry filling into the well in the center.
8. Place the baking sheet in the oven and bake for 20 minutes.
9. Take out the cookies and let cool.
10. You can keep the remaining filling for using it in other recipes.

Pecan Pumpkin Cookies

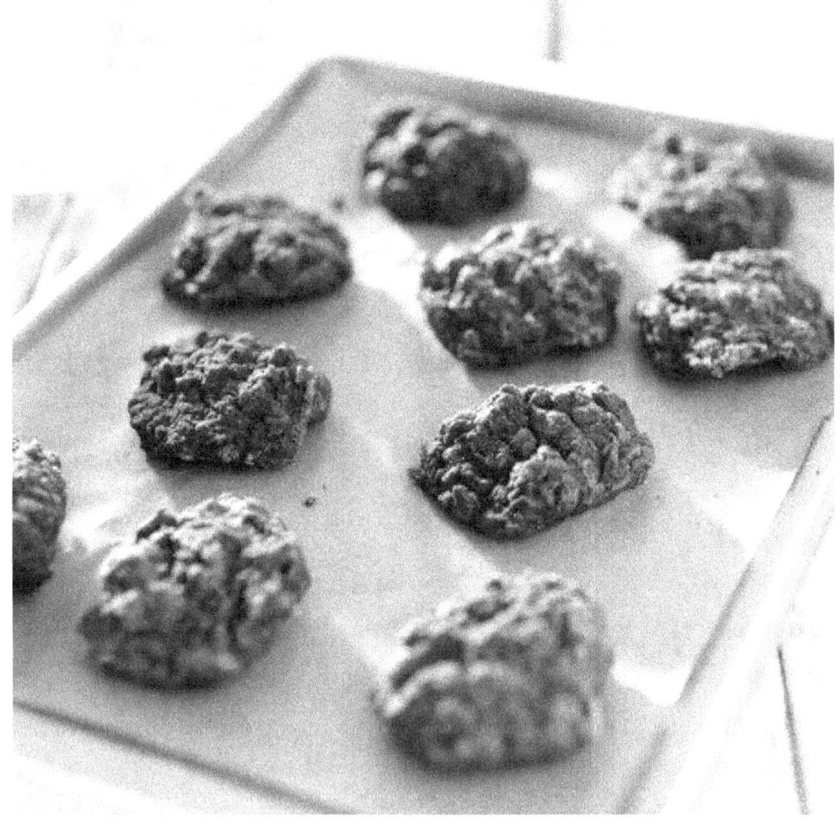

SERVES: 2-3

PREPARATION TIME: 10 minutes

INGREDIENTS:

Pecans 1/3 cup

Almonds ¼ cup

Pitted dates ¾ cup (8 large)

Ground flaxseed ¼ cup

Canned pumpkin 3 tablespoons

Vanilla 1 teaspoon

Pumpkin pie spice 1.5 teaspoon

Cinnamon ½ teaspoon
Salt a pinch
METHOD:

1. Take a baking sheet and line it with parchment paper.
2. Put almonds and pecans in a jar of food processor. Pulse until the mixture forms fine crumbs. Remove and place in a medium bowl.
3. Put dates in the food processor and pulse to make a smooth paste.
4. Return the mixture of processed nuts to the food processor with the dates. Add the remaining ingredients and pulse to combine everything well.
5. Remove the dough and make a large ball. Now, make 8 balls out of the dough and flatten them to make cookies.
6. Refrigerate for a while and serve cold.

Cashew Cardamom Date Balls

When your kids come rushing home from school and ask for something to eat immediately, just ask them to wait for 10 minutes and quickly make them these quick cashew balls. Apart from the health benefits of dates and cashews, these balls taste amazing too.

SERVES: 2-3
PREPARATION TIME: 10 minutes
INGREDIENTS:
Cashews 1 cup
Pitted medjool dates 1 cup
Orange zest 1 orange
Cardamom ¼ teaspoon
Coconut flakes 1/3 cup
METHOD:

1. Leaving coconut aside, put all the ingredients in the food processor. Pulse until all the components are combined well.
2. Make balls of the mixture about the size of a tablespoon.
3. Roll the balls in coconut flakes. If you find that the coconut flakes are not sticking to the balls, you can use a little water to coat them.
4. Serve fresh.

Carrot Cake Cookies

The goodness of carrots with the amazing taste of chocolate is just what you need during winter. Have these cookies with a glass of organic milk or a smoothie, and your healthy tasty breakfast is done!

SERVES: 4-5

PREPARATION TIME: 50 minutes

INGREDIENTS:

Shredded carrots 2 large

Coconut sugar 1 cup

Coconut oil, melted 1 cup

Whisked eggs 2

Vanilla extract 1 teaspoon

Coconut flour 1 cup

Tapioca flour ½ cup

Pumpkin pie spice ½ teaspoon

Chocolate chunks 1 cup

METHOD:

1. Preheat the oven to a temperature of 350 degrees Fahrenheit.
2. Take a bowl large enough to accommodate carrots, coconut oil, coconut sugar, vanilla extract and eggs. Whisk the ingredients and combine them well.
3. Add tapioca flour, coconut flour, salt and pumpkin spice. Mix them and combine.
4. Add chocolate chunks in the mixture and fold them in. You might find the dough a little dry and hard. The cookies will be fine after baking.
5. Take a baking sheet and line it with parchment paper.
6. Take an ice cream scoop and take out 12-13 scoops of the dough onto the baking dish. Press down the cookies using your fingers.

7. Put the baking tray in the oven and cook for 35-40 minutes. The cookies should be cooked through.

Ginger Cookies

Ginger gives cookies a deliciously warm, tangy flavor. If you are a fan of ginger, this recipe will be a winner for you.

SERVES: 12

PREPARATION TIME: 50 minutes

INGREDIENTS:

Almond flour 1.5 cups

Softened coconut oil 2 tablespoons

Maple syrup ¼ cup

Blackstrap molasses 1 tablespoon

Ground ginger 2 teaspoons

Sea salt 1/8 teaspoon

Baking soda ¼ teaspoon

METHOD:

1. Put all the ingredients in a bowl. Mix to combine them well.
2. Refrigerate the mixture for 30 minutes. It should become firm before you take it out of the fridge.
3. Preheat the oven to a temperature of 350 degrees Fahrenheit.
4. Take a baking sheet and line it with parchment paper.
5. Scoop out balls of dough onto the baking dish. You can flatten the balls using a fork till you reach the desired thickness.
6. Put the baking sheet in the oven and cook for 8-10 minutes. They will become firm around the edges, but will remain soft in the center.
7. Take out the sheet and let them cool for 10 minutes.
8. Transfer the cookies on a cooling rack and then serve.

Pumpkin Pie Cookies

These cookies might become your favorite once you have them. Have them for breakfast or after lunch, the soft cookies will please you anytime.

SERVES: 24
PREPARATION TIME: 25 minutes
INGREDIENTS:
Almond butter, creamy 1 cup
Pumpkin puree ½ cup
Maple syrup ¼ cup
Pumpkin pie spice 2 teaspoons
Sea salt ¼ teaspoon
Dark chocolate chips ½ cup
METHOD:

1. Preheat the oven to a temperature of 350 degrees Fahrenheit.
2. Take a baking sheet and line it with parchment paper.
3. In a medium sized bowl, put all the ingredients and mix them to form a thick batter.
4. Put in the chocolate chips and fold them into the batter.
5. Since you are not putting eggs in this recipe, you can taste it to test at any point of time and adjust the ingredients accordingly.
6. Drop a tablespoon or a scoop of the batter for each cookie onto the baking sheet. Use a wet fork to press the cookies down a little.
7. Bake them for 12-15 minutes until you see the edges becoming golden.
8. Take the sheet out of the oven and let cool.
9. Chill the cookies before serving.

<u>Banana Bacon Cookies</u>

Bananas make these cookies melt in your mouth. The softness is unparalleled to any other cookies. Moreover, there is bacon to enhance the taste.

SERVES: 3-4
PREPARATION TIME: 30 minutes
INGREDIENTS:
Mashed bananas 2 small
Sunflower seed butter 1 cup
Honey ½ cup
Whisked egg 1
Vanilla extract 1 teaspoon
Cinnamon ¼ teaspoon
Baking soda ½ teaspoon
Baking powder ½ teaspoon
Salt a pinch
Chocolate chips ½ cup
Cooked and diced bacon 3 strips

METHOD:

1. Preheat the oven to a temperature of 350 degrees Fahrenheit.
2. Take a baking sheet and line it with parchment paper.
3. Take a medium sized bowl and put in butter, banana, egg, honey, and vanilla. Mix them well.
4. Add baking powder, baking soda, salt and cinnamon. Mix well.
5. Put bacon and chocolate chips into the mixture and fold them through properly.
6. Scoop out tablespoons of batter onto the baking sheet. Leave

some room between each cookie to allow them to spread out. The batter will make about 12 cookies.

7. Put the tray in the oven and cook for 20 minutes. Take it out and let cool.
8. Serve.

<u>Macadamia Nut Cookies</u>

Macadamia nuts always taste good, and they're especially yummy when combined with chocolate, as in this recipe.

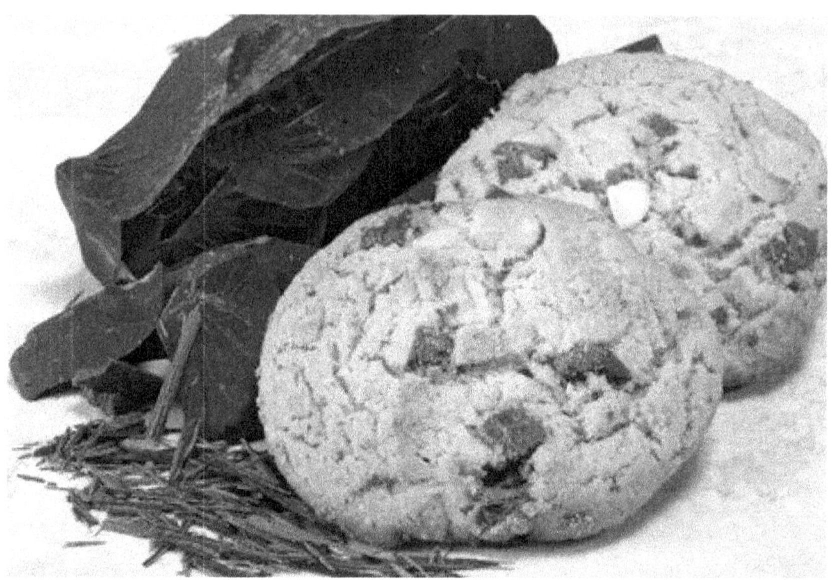

SERVES: 3-4

PREPARATION TIME: 40 minutes

INGREDIENTS:

Almond flour 2.5 cups

Coconut flour 2 tablespoons

Shredded coconut, unsweetened 2/3 cups

Baking soda 1 teaspoon

Melted coconut oil ½ cup

Melted raw honey ¼ cup

Whisked eggs 3

Vanilla extract 1 tablespoon

Macadamia nuts 2/3 cup

Chocolate chips 2/3 cup

Sea salt ¼ teaspoon
METHOD:

1. Preheat the oven to a temperature of 350 degrees Fahrenheit.
2. Take a baking sheet and line it with aluminum sheets.
3. In a medium sized bowl, mix coconut flour, almond flour, sea salt, baking soda and shredded coconut.
4. Take another bowl to mix together vanilla extract, eggs, honey and coconut oil. Pour the mixture into the other bowl.
5. Add chocolate chips and macadamia nuts and fold them in the mixture.
6. Make balls about the size of 2 tablespoons of batter. Position these balls on the baking sheet and press them down using your hand.
7. Place the cookies in the oven and cook for 18-20 minutes. Check after 16 minutes that the bottom of the cookies are not overcooking or burning.
8. Let them cool after you take them out.
9. Serve and enjoy!

<u>Orange Blossom Cookies</u>

The tangy taste of oranges in the cookies is just so awesome. The freshness of the orange juice remains intact even after baking.

SERVES: 3-4

PREPARATION TIME: 30 minutes

INGREDIENTS:

Almond flour 3 cups

Coconut flour ¼ cup

Melted coconut oil 1/3 cup

Navel orange zest 1 large

Vanilla extract 1 tablespoon

Baking soda, aluminum free ½ teaspoon

Sea salt a pinch

Honey, local, raw 1/3 cup

Orange juice 1/3 cup (from half navel orange)

METHOD:

1. Preheat the oven to a temperature of 350 degrees Fahrenheit.
2. Take a baking sheet and line it with parchment paper.
3. Put all the ingredients in a glass bowl and mix them using a pastry blender.
4. Make a large dough ball of the mixture and place it on a piece of wax paper. Refrigerate the dough for 15 minutes.
5. Make 1.5 inch sized balls out of the dough and position them on the sheet.
6. Press down the balls using a wet fork. You can also make a pattern of cross hatching with the fork.
7. Put the baking sheet in the oven and bake the cookies for 15 minutes. The top crust of the cookies should become golden brown.
8. Take the sheet out of the oven and let cool.

9. Serve and enjoy.

Sunflower Cookies

The visual appeal as well as taste of these cookies puts them in a class of their own. The sunflower seeds and butter give these Paleo cookies a completely unique taste. Serve them with a cup of coffee and enjoy the delicacy.

SERVES: 3-4

PREPARATION TIME: 30 minutes

INGREDIENTS (for cookies):

Coconut flour 6 tablespoons

Sunflower seed butter/ nut butter ½ cup

Coconut sugar 2/3 cup

Melted coconut oil 1/3 cup

Egg 1

INGREDIENTS (for decoration):

Sunflower seeds 2 tablespoons

Dark chocolate chips (optional) 12

METHOD:

1. Preheat the oven to a temperature of 350 degrees Fahrenheit.
2. Take a baking sheet and line it with parchment paper or grease the sheet.
3. In a large bowl, put egg, sunflower seed butter, coconut sugar, coconut oil and coconut flour. Mix well to combine the ingredients.
4. Keep the dough in the freezer for 10-12 minutes. This makes the dough less sticky and the cookies also spread less after freezing.
5. Put the chocolate chips and sunflower seeds in a small bowl.
6. Take the dough out from the freezer and make 12 balls out of it. Place these balls on the baking sheet. Flatten them gently.
7. Push a chocolate chip in the center of each cookie. You can

avoid chocolate chips if you do not like them with sunflower seeds. Now decorate the cookies with sunflower seeds. Push the seeds gently into the cookies

8. Bake them for 12 minutes. Take the baking sheet out of the oven and let cool.

9. Serve at room temperature.

<u>Lazy Espresso Cookies</u>

Sometimes, you just do not have time for a proper meal during busy hours in the office. A quick shot of espresso cookies is a great way to energize you when you need a pick-me-up at the office. Just grab one of these cookies if you didn't have time to have lunch today!

SERVES: 4-5

PREPARATION TIME: 30 minutes

INGREDIENTS:

Almond flour 2 cups

Baking soda ¼ teaspoon

Salt a pinch

Cinnamon 2 dashes

Espresso powder 1-2 tablespoons

Coconut powder or shredded coconut, unsweetened ½ cup

Coconut oil 1/3 cup

Maple syrup ¼ cup

Vanilla extract 1 teaspoon

Coconut milk 1 tablespoon

Chocolate chips ¾ cup

METHOD:

1. Preheat the oven to a temperature of 350 degrees Fahrenheit.
2. Take a baking sheet and line it with parchment paper.
3. In a medium sized bowl, put all the ingredients and combine them well.
4. Add chocolate chips and fold them in the batter.
5. Make balls of this dough about the size of a heaping tablespoon.
6. Place the balls in the baking sheet and flatten them using your hands. Leave a gap of about one inch between each cookie to allow them some room to spread.

7. Put the baking tray in the oven and cook for 12-15 minutes.
8. Remove the tray from the oven and let it cool for 2 minutes.
9. Transfer the cookies on the wire rack and let cool for a while.
10. Serve warm or at room temperature.

Avocado Double Chocolate Cookies

The earthy and fresh flavor of avocado seems to go with anything. Even if you combine avocado with cookies, the texture and taste comes out really well. Enjoy these cookies and save some for later as well.

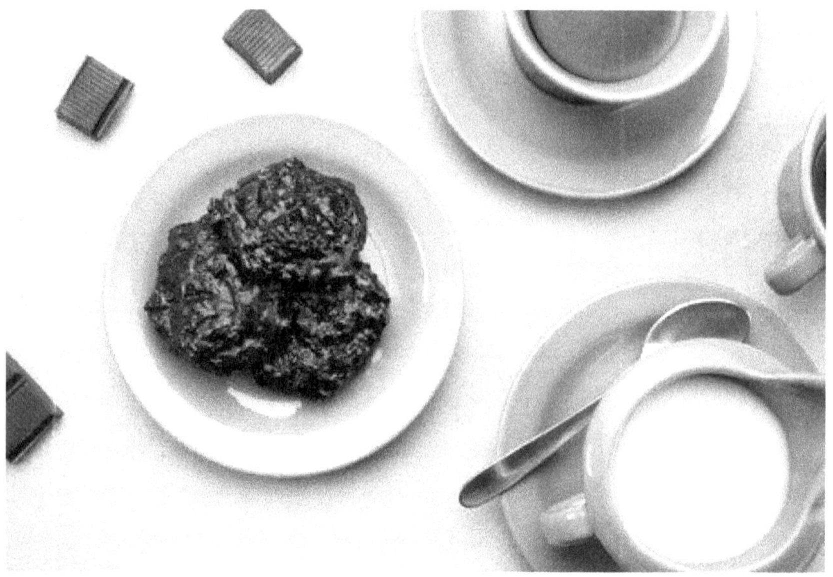

SERVES: 4-5

PREPARATION TIME: 25 minutes

INGREDIENTS:

Baking soda ½ teaspoon

Water 1 tablespoon

Avocado, very ripe 1

Maple syrup ¼ cup

Egg 1

Cocoa powder ½ cup

Dark chocolate, unsweetened, chopped 1 ounce

METHOD:

1. Preheat the oven to a temperature of 350 degrees Fahrenheit.
2. Take a baking sheet and line it with parchment paper and keep aside.
3. In a small bowl, mix baking soda with water and set aside.
4. Using a hand blender, whip avocado properly. Add maple syrup and continue whipping to achieve a smooth mixture.
5. Add egg and whisk again.
6. Add cocoa powder gradually and continue mixing on a medium speed of the blender.
7. Once you are done adding the ingredients mentioned, turn on the high speed and mix well. Mix baking soda mixture into this mixture and blend it well with everything else.
8. Add chopped chocolate. Stir well to combine the chocolate. The dough will be soft in texture.
9. Using an ice-cream scoop, scoop out two tablespoons sized dough on the baking sheet. Keep a gap of at least 2 inches in between the cookies. Flatten them using the back side of a spoon.
10. Bake the cookies for 8-10 minutes. It is fine if they look slightly underdone.
11. Take the baking sheet out of the oven and let it cool slightly.
12. Transfer the cookies on a wire rack and let them cool properly.
13. Serve.

Sandwich Cookies

This last recipe of the book is so worth the extra effort. You only need an ice cream maker at home. If you do not have it, do not worry. You can make normal cream using simple tools. Just go ahead and make these sandwich cookies. Your entire family is going to love them. Enjoy them in the evening with smoothies or coffee.

SERVES: 4-5
PREPARATION TIME: 25 minutes
INGREDIENTS (for cookies):
Almond flour 2 cups
Salt ½ teaspoon
Baking soda ½ teaspoon
Pumpkin pie spice 1 tablespoon (more for adding sprinkles)
Pumpkin puree ½ cup
Mashed and ripe banana 1 small
Maple syrup ¼ cup
Vanilla extract 1 tablespoon
Coconut oil 1/3 cup
Chocolate chips ½ cup

INGREDIENTS (for cream filling):

Coconut milk 1 can

Pumpkin puree 1 can

Maple syrup ¼ cup

Pumpkin pie spice ½ tablespoon

METHOD (for cookies):

1. Preheat the oven to a temperature of 350 degrees Fahrenheit.
2. Take a baking sheet and line it with parchment paper.
3. Take a large bowl and put baking soda, almond flour, pumpkin pie spice, and salt. Mix the ingredients well.
4. In another bowl, mix mashed banana, pumpkin puree, vanilla extract and maple syrup. Mix these ingredients well and pour them into the other bowl containing dry ingredients.
5. Add coconut oil and mix well to incorporate it with the mixture.
6. Add chocolate chips and fold them in the batter.
7. Scoop out a tablespoonful of batter on the baking sheet for each cookie. Make as many cookies as needed to finish the batter.
8. Sprinkle pumpkin pie spice on top of the cookies.
9. Put the baking sheet in the oven and cook for 25-30 minutes. The cookies will become golden brown.
10. Take the baking sheet out of the oven and let cool.
11. Serve after cooling them.
12. You can store the remaining cookies in the refrigerator in an airtight jar.

METHOD (for cream filling):

1. Put all the ingredients of cream filling into a medium sized bowl, and stir well to combine.
2. Make ice-cream in the ice-cream maker.

ASSEMBLING THE COOKIES:

1. Place a few cookies upside down and put a scoop of cream filling in the center. Top it with another cookie with its bottom facing the cream.
2. Refrigerate for a while and serve. The ice-cream should be placed in the cookies sandwiches while they are still warm. It makes it easy to assemble the cookies.

Conclusion

We hope that you have enjoyed the delicious cookies and desserts in *Gluten Free Paleo Cookies*. You might never have realized that cookies and brownies can be made in so many different ways. There are many options to explore new things with limited ingredients. You do not have to indulge in unhealthy things to savor the taste of some of the best foods in the world.

You can also take your Paleo diet to another level. Host a Paleo party at your place, and tell your friends to come prepared for cooking as well as eating healthy. It is so much fun eating food that you have cooked together with friends. And, this is not just a girls' thing to indulge in; you can call in the guys as well! They should also know about this concept of eating healthily. Convince them to leave the comfort of their beds and come to your place for cooking on a weekend. We are sure that you will all have fun together.

You can also make suitable changes to the recipes mentioned in this book. Just evaluate the changes your additional ingredients will make to the basic recipe. Alternatively, you can substitute one component with another. A small change in a recipe can make a huge difference. But obviously, the change should be positive. You would not like to eat a cookie as hard as stone! Be cautious while baking and the result will definitely be positive.

Go ahead and enjoy the treat of cookies and desserts, guilt-free!

© Copyright 2019_All rights reserved.

<u>Disclaimer</u>:

The information presented in this book represents the views of the publisher as of the date of publication. The publisher reserves the rights to alter update their opinions based on new conditions. This report is for informational purposes only. The author and the publisher do not accept any responsibilities for any liabilities resulting from the use of this information. While every attempt has been made to verify the information provided here, the author and the publisher cannot assume any responsibility for errors, inaccuracies or omissions. Any similarities with people or facts are unintentional.

www.ingramcontent.com/pod-product-compliance
Lightning Source LLC
Chambersburg PA
CBHW071738150726
47998CB00005B/1701